THEN AND THERE SERIES
GENERAL EDITOR
MARJORIE REEVES

A Hundred Years of Medical Care

Second Edition

ALAN DELGADO

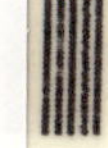

LONGMAN GROUP UK LIMITED
*Longman House,
Burnt Mill, Harlow, Essex, CM20 2JE, England
and Associated Companies throughout the world*

*First published 1970
Second edition 1982
Fourth impression 1987*

ISBN 0 582 22054 8

*Produced by Longman Group (FE) Ltd
Printed in Hong Kong*

Acknowledgements We are grateful to the following for permission to reproduce copyright material. Author's agents and Willian Heinemann Ltd. for an extract from *Dr. Bradley Remembers* by Francis Brett Young; The Proprietors of *The Guardian* for a letter from Charles R. H. Pickard from issue dated 15th February 1968; Pitman Medical Publishing Co. Ltd. for extracts from *Six Disciples of Florence Nightingale* by Z. Cope; Routledge & Kegan Paul Ltd. for an extract from *Confessions of an English Doctor* (anon.).
We have been unable to trace the copyright holder of *Diary of a Medical Student* by S. Taylor, and would appreciate any information that would enable us to do so.
The author is indebted to friends in the medical profession who read the typescript and made helpful comments; to The Wellcome Historical Medical Library, and to the authors of these books: *Florence Nightingale* by Cecil Woodham Smith (Constable), *Florence Nightingale's Nurses* by Lucy Seymer (Pitman Medical), *Elizabeth Garrett Anderson* by Jo Manton (Methuen), *A History of the Nursing Profession* by Brian Abel-Smith (Heinemann). The extract from Rebecca Strong's *Reminiscences* in Chapter 3 is quoted by permission of John Menzies (Holdings) Ltd.
For permission to reproduce photographs we are grateful to the following: Sir Colin Anderson, page 43 *right;* Associated Newspapers Ltd, page 77; the Trustees of the British Museum, page 21 *left;* Elizabeth Garrett Anderson Hospital, pages 35 and 43 *left;* King's College Hospital Medical School, page 71; *Illustrated London News*, pages 12, 15 and 16; Henry Grant, page 81; the Matron of St Thomas' Hospital and the Greater London Record Office, page 21; the Trustees of the National Portrait Gallery, pages 4 and 14; *Punch*, pages 36, 46, 48 and 74; Queen Victoria Hospital East Grinstead, page 59; The Royal Free Hospital School of Medicine, page 39; the Trustees of the Tate Gallery, page 51; Sir Harry Verney, Bart., page 25; the Wellcome Trustees, pages 18, 64 and 65. The top photograph on page 58 is taken from E J Dennison's *A Cottage Hospital Grows Up* Anthony Blond, by courtesy of the author and publisher. Cover: BOC Limited, D. Fullerton, The Wellcome Trustees.

Contents

To the Reader

This book is about the care of the sick, and the people who brought about changes in that sphere from approximately 1846 to 1948 when the National Health Service began. After nearly forty years what has the Health Service achieved and what are the problems? The final chapter discusses them and shows what is now done to prevent illness.

If you had lived in Queen Victoria's day or any time up to the outbreak of the First World War in 1914, how would you have been treated if you were ill? As you will find out, it depended on whether you were rich or poor.

The medical profession in the last century was a man's world. It was unthinkable that a woman could become a doctor, or that a nurse should be other than a slut who did the dirty tasks and was given an occasional swig of beer for any particularly unpleasant duty. Yet it was two women who changed all that.

Florence Nightingale was one. She appears often in this book. The picture of her moving with her lamp silently amongst the wounded soldiers in the Crimean War may be romantic, but in her frail body burned the crusading spirit and she had a mind as sharp as steel. It was due to her that nurses were trained and gained a better position. She was interested in everything to do with medical care and had strong views on it all. As you will discover, Miss Nightingale did not mince words. She feared nobody.

The other woman was Elizabeth Garrett who was determined to become a doctor. Anyone with less courage would have been put off by the obstacles in her way, but because she struggled on so obstinately, women were able to enter that all-male preserve – the medical profession.

Both these fighters were stifled by the Victorian attitude towards women. In those days it was difficult for women to break away from the pattern of life laid down for them and to which they were expected to conform. If they wanted to do something else with their lives everyone – including their families – was against them. They could not 'demonstrate' with others of a like mind because they were isolated in a tightly-knit family. They had to go it alone. You will read of the hardships of these two women, yet, at a time when people died young, they lived to a ripe old age, showered with honours by those (mostly men) who had opposed them.

There were discoveries which improved medical care – the application of *anaesthetics** by James Young Simpson and the introduction of *antiseptic precautions* by Joseph Lister. It was due to the work of these two men that suffering was lessened, the death rate fell and the operating theatre ceased to be a slaughter house.

In more recent times you will see how medical care became the responsibility of the State, so that everybody now has a right to medical attention without worrying about how they are going to pay for it.

You will hear about 'preventive medicine'. That means, quite simply, preventing illness by regular medical examinations such as are given in schools and industry, changing living conditions for the better so that the causes of *epidemics* are removed, for example by being inoculated or vaccinated to prevent one getting a particular illness.

You who have been brought up since the days of the National Health Service may find it hard to believe what you read about medical care before that time. Here is part of a letter written to a National newspaper in 1968 by a man of 95 years of age:

> 'I had my tonsils out when I was nineteen. I stood opposite [the doctor] and he showed me the instrument he was

*Words printed in *italics* are explained in the Glossary, p. 88.

going to use and I handled it and saw how it worked. There was no anaesthetic, no hospital, no nurse. I opened my mouth wide . . . the cutting end of the instrument was fitted over one tonsil, and the doctor pushed the cutter through the tonsil and cut it off. It was certainly a painful ordeal, and I was given a few minutes to recover, and then the same process was repeated at the other side. After a short while, to attend to the bleeding, I walked home (about a mile).'

This must have happened in 1892.

NOTE: In the text amounts of money are written in the old pounds, shillings and pence (£ *s d*). In today's money one old shilling is worth five new pence (5p). There were twenty shillings in £1 and twelve old pence made one shilling.

1 *Florence Nightingale's Early Days*

You may have visited Chatsworth, the stately home of the Duke of Devonshire. In August 1842 the Duke of Devonshire at that time invited wealthy friends to Chatsworth to meet His Royal Highness the Duke of Sussex, sixth son of George III who reigned from 1760 to 1820.

Chatsworth was a wonderful sight that night. The house was brilliantly illuminated in honour of the royal guest. It was a gala occasion – brilliant jewellery, beautiful dresses, the grandest clothes. Joseph Paxton, head gardener at Chatsworth and later the designer of the Crystal Palace, had built a large conservatory in the Park. It covered an acre of ground, and for those who could not walk from the house to the conservatory, an omnibus was ready to take them.

One of the guests was a young woman of twenty-two. She should have been enjoying herself, but she was unhappy at the splendour and grandeur of the occasion. The devoted young man at her side who wanted to marry her might not have existed. Her thoughts were elsewhere. She had become aware of the suffering and misery in the world outside Chatsworth, and she wanted to do something about it. The young woman's name was Florence Nightingale.

Her family were wealthy and had houses in London, Hampshire and at Lea Hurst in Derbyshire, some twelve miles as the crow flies from Chatsworth. The nearest village to Lea Hurst was Holloway, and there Florence Nightingale had seen with her own eyes the poverty and sickness that existed. She wrote: 'My mind is absorbed with the idea of the sufferings of man, it *besets* me behind and before, a very one-sided view, but I can

CHOLERA.

THE

DUDLEY BOARD OF HEALTH,

HEREBY GIVE NOTICE, THAT IN CONSEQUENCE OF THE

Church-yards at Dudley

Being so full, no one who has died of the CHOLERA will be permitted to be buried after *SUNDAY* next, (To-morrow) in either of the Burial Grounds of *St. Thomas's*, or *St. Edmund's*, in this Town.

All Persons who die from CHOLERA, must for the future be buried in the Church-yard at Netherton

BOARD of HEALTH, DUDLEY.

A grim notice displayed in the early part of Queen Victoria's reign. Cholera was an infectious disease which killed thousands in overcrowded cities

hardly see anything else and all that poets sing of the glories of this world seems to me untrue.'

How had the suffering and misery which so disturbed her come about? Victoria had been Queen since 1837 and was still in her early twenties. By the time she died in 1901 there were twice as many people living in England and Wales as there had been fifty years before. In that period Britain was covered by a network of railways, new industry in Lancashire and the Black Country developed quickly, the coal mines and the ironworks of the north-west and the Clyde flourished. Towns, to accommodate the thousands of workers, were built in haste and without thought. Rows and rows of *squat* little houses (they are there today) were erected in the shadows of huge industrial works. Smoke belched from tall chimneys; there was grit, dirt and fumes which the inhabitants of the towns were unable to escape.

People in the country and from Ireland and Scotland poured into the towns to find work. Under such living conditions disease and epidemics – including two dangerous fevers, typhus and cholera – were commonplace. *Sanitation* was hardly thought about. Solid filth formed a crust on rivers. Little, if anything, was done about drainage.

This was the world that surrounded Florence Nightingale, but she was not part of it. She had been born in Italy in Florence (hence her name) on 12 May 1820, and she had a sister, Parthenope, born in Naples the previous year. Her parents, William Edward Nightingale and his beautiful wife Fanny, were wealthy and clever. Florence was brought up in the family houses in Hampshire and Derbyshire where she and her sister were taught music and art by a governess, and were instructed by their father in Latin, German, French and Italian.

For Florence it was – or should have been – a secure, calm childhood with loving companionship from her family. Her mother was a very energetic woman who never seemed to weary; her father was the opposite – clever, kindly but lazy and reluctant to make a decision or act on one. Florence had little in common with her sister: Parthenope was untidy and wild; Florence was the opposite – neat and tidy in mind and person.

Although there was all the comfort that money could buy, Florence felt stifled. It was like living in a hot-house. There was nobody to whom she felt she could talk or confide in. The only way she could express herself was on paper, and she was always writing what she called 'private notes'. Sometimes she wrote pages and pages; on other occasions a single sentence was enough. She would never throw away a piece of paper if it could be used for writing on. She hoarded every scrap and these private notes appeared on the odd piece of blotting paper, the back of a calendar or in the margin of a letter.

When Florence was sixteen and her sister seventeen, it was decided they must follow the custom of wealthy young ladies of that time and be 'launched' into society. This meant entertaining on a grand scale – dinners, parties, dances. The Nightingale country house in Hampshire – Embley – where the 'launching' party was to take place was considered too small.

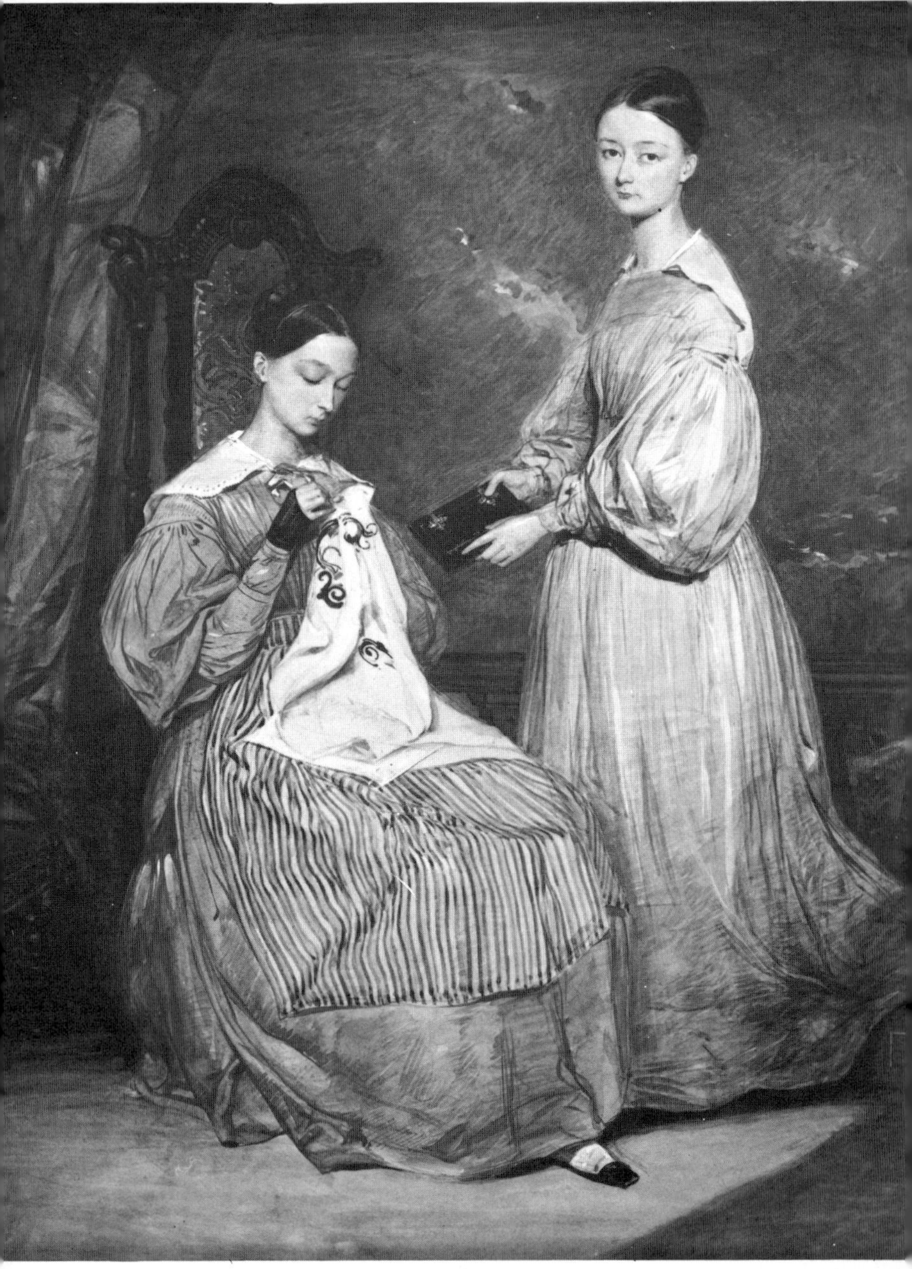

Six more bedrooms were to be added, new kitchens installed and the whole house completely redecorated. In the middle of these important preparations, Florence heard, for the first time, the voice of God. In a note Florence wrote, 'On February 7th 1837 God spoke to me and called me to His service'.

What service Florence was expected to render to God had not been made clear to her. But she now knew that she was to serve God in some way, and she was content. The 'stifled' feeling left her. She now had faith and felt sure that God would speak to her again.

Seven months later the Nightingale family boarded a boat at Southampton and sailed for Le Havre in France. Mrs Nightingale took her maid, the girls were in charge of a nurse. There was also a *courier*. A continental tour, Mr Nightingale reckoned, would be just the thing while the house in Hampshire was being enlarged and redecorated. Besides, it would be good for the girls; they could speak the languages their father had taught them, go to parties, listen to music, visit art galleries and buy clothes in Paris.

The European tour lasted eighteen months. Mrs Nightingale was delighted with her daughters. She was particularly pleased with Florence who had blossomed in society and had a promising future. The alterations to Embley, the house in Hampshire, would soon be completed. In the meantime, the girls would stay in London and be 'presented' to Queen Victoria at Buckingham Palace, as was customary in that social circle. But what were Florence's feelings? She had enjoyed herself abroad. She loved all the pleasures that had come her way, she delighted in meeting people, she was enchanted with the foreign countries she had visited. God had not spoken to her again. In fact, God had not been foremost in her mind – she was too much in love with life on earth. But just before she left Paris she wrote one of her notes. In it she expressed a wish to be worthy of becoming one of God's servants. To achieve this, she realised she must overcome her 'desire to shine in society'.

Opposite: *the young Florence Nightingale (seated) with her sister Parthenope*

Nevertheless the gay, social life continued and Florence became more and more impatient of it. Her one wish, as she wrote in later years, was to have 'a necessary occupation, something to fill and employ all my *faculties*'. She also wrote, 'O weary days! O evenings that seem never to end! For how many long years I have watched that drawing-room clock and thought it would never reach ten!' At ten o'clock the family went to bed.

In 1845, when she was twenty-five, she made an astounding suggestion to her parents. It was that she should be allowed to nurse for a few months at the nearby hospital in Salisbury. Her parents' reply can be imagined. It was unthinkable, they said. Hospitals were the most dreadful places and no well-brought-up girl could possibly go near one! 'I shall never do anything, and am worse than dust and nothing,' Florence lamented. 'What have I done in this world and what have I done this last fortnight?' she wrote in her diary on 7 July 1847. 'I have read to Papa [and] Mamma. Learnt seven tunes by heart. Written various letters. Ridden with Papa. Paid eight visits. Done Company [meaning entertained visitors]. And that is all.

Her family worried about her. She had become bad-tempered, out of sorts – nothing like the Florence they knew. Where had they gone wrong? They had loved her and given her happiness and security. Marriage? Yes, she had thought about marriage, but if she married she could not serve God in the way He wanted. She became unwell. Her mother fussed around her. 'Oh, if one has but a toothache,' Florence wrote, 'what remedies are invented! What carriages, horses, ponies, journeys, doctors, *chaperones*, are urged on one; but if it is something the matter with the MIND . . . it is neither believed nor understood.'

It was during this period that she decided to study. She would learn all there was to know about hospitals, sanitation and the treatment of the sick. It all had to be done in secrecy. She would get up at dawn, throw a shawl round her shoulders, and privately in her bedroom would study books, pamphlets and reports from all over the world. The candle-light flickered as this young woman read and made notes. Then, when it was time to dress, she would hide her books away. A short time afterwards she would take her place at the family breakfast table.

But in 1851 Florence had her way. With the help of friends her parents were persuaded to allow her to work at the Kaiserswerth Institute in Germany, a hospital with a hundred beds and opportunities for training. The staff consisted of deaconesses, and life there was very hard. The food was of the simplest. Mrs Nightingale had given in to Florence's request with bad grace. It was not what she had hoped for her daughter. She must have been astonished to receive from Kaiserswerth this letter from Florence:

> 'Until yesterday I never had time even to send my things to the wash. We have ten minutes for each of our meals, of which we have four. We get up at 5; breakfast $\frac{1}{4}$ before 6. The patients dine at 11; the Sisters at 12. We drink tea (i.e. a drink made of ground rye) between 2 and 3, broths at 12 and 7; bread at the two former, vegetables at 12. Several evenings in the week we collect in the Great Hall for a bible lesson . . .
>
> 'I find the deepest interest in everything here and am so well in body and mind. This is life. Now I know what it is to live and to love life, and really I should be sorry now to leave life. I wish for no other earth, no other world than this.'

She remained at Kaiserswerth for about four months. Her family could never forgive her. In October 1851 she joined her mother and sister at Cologne in order to return to England. 'They would hardly speak to me,' she wrote later. 'I was treated as if I had come from committing a crime.'

2 *Journey to the Crimea*

On 9 October 1854 the butler employed by the Nightingale family placed 'The Times' of that day on the breakfast table so that it was ready for the master of the house to read when he came down. 'The Times' was read by many wealthy and influential families, and that particular issue contained some very disturbing news about the war in the Crimea which had been raging since March.

The Crimean War was between Russia (not the Russia we know today but as it was then, ruled by a *Tsar*) on the one side, and England, France and Turkey on the other. War in such distant parts did not affect the lives of those living in England. There was no danger of air raids or invasion. The shops were stocked with the usual luxuries. Life went on very much as before. The Royal Navy ruled the seas and the British Army was unbeatable. Were not the British to thrill a few days later at news of the Charge of the Light Brigade at the Battle of Balaclava?

The disturbing news in 'The Times' on 9 October was from the newspaper's correspondent in Constantinople drawing attention to the appalling sufferings of the British Army.

> 'It is with feelings of surprise and anger that the public will learn that no sufficient preparations have been made for the proper care of the wounded. Not only are there not sufficient surgeons . . . not only are there no *dressers* and nurses . . . but what will be said when it is known that there is not even linen to make bandages for the wounded? Not only are men kept, in some cases, for a week without the hand of a medical man coming near their wounds; not

only are they left to expire in agony, unheeded and shaken off . . . but now it is found that the commonest appliances of a workhouse sick-ward are wanting, and that men must die through the medical staff of the British Army having forgotten that old rags are necessary for the *dressing* of wounds.

And so it continued, imploring action to be taken and putting the blame on the Government 'to make inquiries into the conduct of those who have so greatly neglected their duty'.

'The Times' was an influential newspaper and the nation was disturbed at the revelations. It was embarrassing too, that our allies the French had excellent medical arrangements assisted by some fifty Sisters of Charity who made excellent nurses.

'Why have we no Sisters of Charity?' wrote somebody in anger to 'The Times'. 'There are a number of able-bodied and tender-hearted English women who would joyfully and with *alacrity* go out to devote themselves to nursing the sick and wounded if they could be placed under proper protection.'

Florence Nightingale was just the woman to leap to such a challenge. With the help of the Government she searched Great Britain for nurses. They were not easy to come by. Nursing was not a profession and the women who came forward were, in some cases, a very rough lot. Young women were not acceptable as there would be dangers. Nevertheless she collected together thirty-eight, of whom twenty-four were nuns (Roman Catholic or Anglican), the others of no particular religion, except perhaps to worship the intoxicating content of a bottle. The sisters and nuns were more concerned with healing the souls of the patients; the nurses saw their work as restoring the bodily health of the sick. 'Excellent self-devoted women', wrote Florence Nightingale of some of the nuns, 'fit more for heaven than a hospital, they flit about like angels without hands among the patients and soothe their souls while they leave their bodies dirty and neglected.'

Most of the nurses were stout and elderly which prompted Florence Nightingale to write from the Crimea that if more

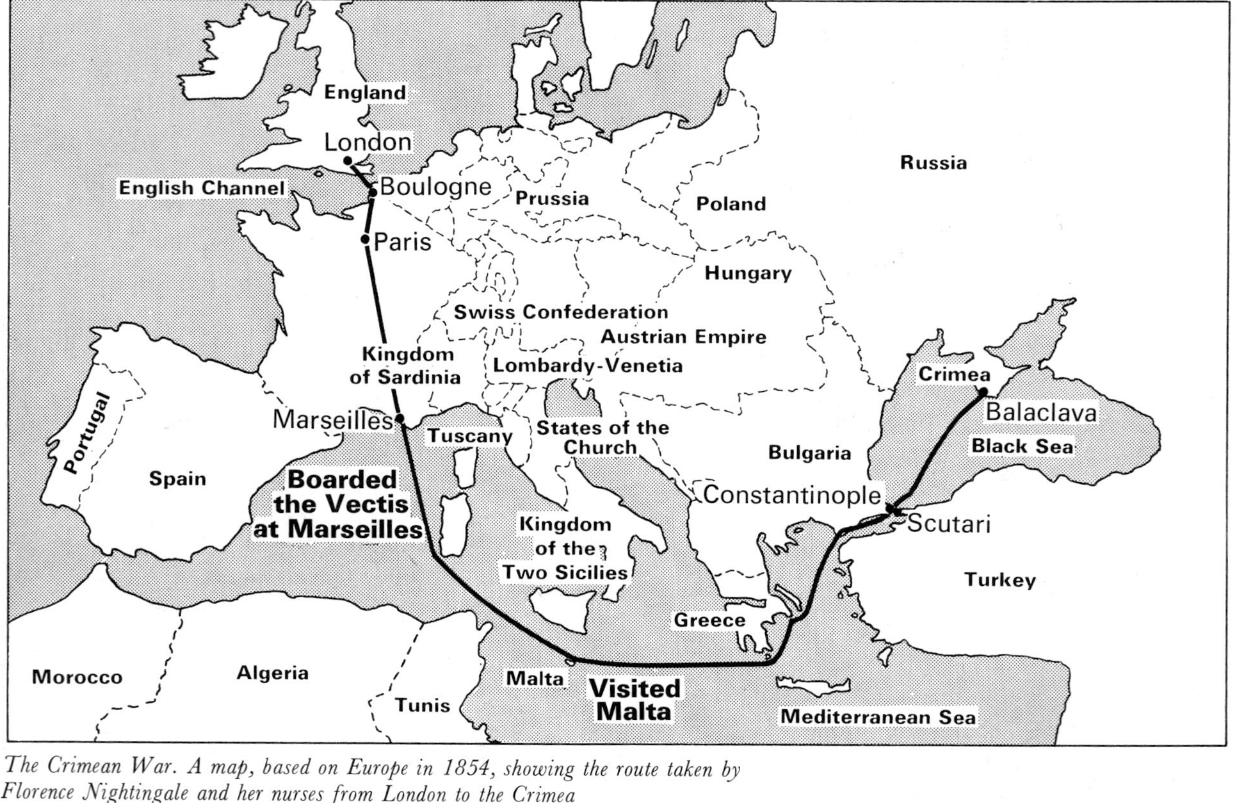

The Crimean War. A map, based on Europe in 1854, showing the route taken by Florence Nightingale and her nurses from London to the Crimea

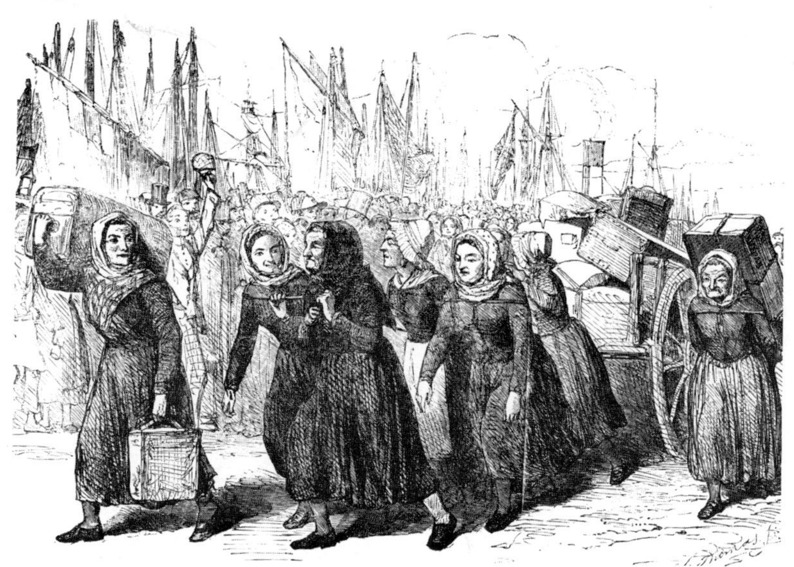

Journey to the Crimea. Porter-women at Boulogne carrying the nurses' baggage

nurses were sent to her, 'fat drunken old dames of fourteen stone and over must be barred, the provision of bedsteads is not strong enough'.

Each nurse was to be paid 12*s* to 14*s* a week, plus their *keep* and uniform. The pay was increased after a certain time if conduct was good. Each nurse had to sign a document agreeing to obey Miss Nightingale's orders. Each nurse was to bring her own underclothes, four cotton night-caps, one cotton umbrella and a carpet-bag. No frills like ribbons were permitted. Rules about what, and how much they drank, were strict and the necessary standards of good behaviour were explained to them.

This assorted collection of women suffered dreadful hardship on the journey. Let Sister Sarah Terrot (an Anglican nun) tell the story of the voyage to Scutari. First she tells how, on 21 October 1854 she, with the other nurses, dressed simply in black, assembled at 6 o'clock in the morning at London Bridge Station. Florence Nightingale had gone ahead to Paris. As the boat left Folkestone for Boulogne 'the crowd, knowing our destination gave us three hearty cheers'. Sister Sarah was a good sailor, but 'the rest of the party, with the nuns and nurses all proved themselves unable to withstand the disastrous effects of a swell in the English Channel'.

At last, though, 'we stood rather giddy on the pier at Boulogne. We walked to the hotel, where a very tasteful display of French cooking awaited us, for which the host refused payment. The poor merry-hearted porter-women also insisted on carrying our luggage without payment.'

The party sailed from Marseilles on a ship called the 'Vectis':

> 'When we got on deck we found ourselves in a little steamer, and were at once introduced to our quarters, which were in the fore-cabin where there were berths for forty, which we fully occupied. They were divided into little recesses nearest the forepart of the boat, of course the most confined and farthest from fresh air, though the more retired. The nuns had a little division for themselves at the foot of the cabin stairs. The nurses lay in between. In bad weather, the nuns were best off for air, though they paid for this advantage by having a double allowance of water which the boat constantly shipped, and which washed over the deck and came down the cabin stairs. Till overcome by sickness, Sister Mary de Gonzaga was kept pretty busy *swabbing* up. Miss Nightingale being a very bad sailor, retired as soon as we got on board.'

At first the sea was calm, but the 'Vectis' was designed for speed rather than heavy going. They called at Malta and those who felt well enough went ashore sightseeing. Under male supervision the travellers (the nuns dressed in black or white) were assembled–'black sisters in front, white sisters in rear, nurses intermediate'. Like that they marched everywhere the gentleman in charge 'running on before and chatting to every respectable person he met, and announcing to them our meaning: "Nuns, ladies and nurses going to nurse the soldiers of the British Army in the Crimea".'

After leaving Malta the 'Vectis' was tossed like a cork in the rough seas:

'I sat listening to the whistling wind, praying the Lord God Almighty to grant us a quiet night and a Christian end. A little after midnight the noise increased, and one wakeful timid nurse rose and went to the bottom of the stairs. I begged her to sit down quietly, but she would not, and soon a fearful noise began on deck, as if the men were dragging chains. The poor nurse thought this preliminary to the sailors escaping and leaving us to be lost, and she uttered a fearful shriek and then a burst of wild cries for "Mercy this once, only this once!" The nurses being roused from sleep, took up the cry and "Mercy, mercy, Lord, have mercy," resounded on all sides as they hurriedly arose and begun to dress. In vain I tried to quiet them.'

Calm was eventually restored and in the early morning Sister Sarah visited her companions.

'I found Sister Bertha very sick and cheerful and uncomplaining, Sister Ethelreda suffering from exhaustion and want of air. Clara lay on the wet floor, whither she had moved to give Sister Ethelreda more breathing space, and there she lay on the floor, soaking up to the neck, (in sea water happily), day after day, without food and almost without air, till really speechless and half-dead. The sea was still washing the deck and gently pouring into our cabin. . . . It was a dismal scene, the dark wet cabin with one miserable swinging light, just enough to show the sick lying about in every direction. In their own cabin at the bottom of the stairs lay the pale picturesque Sister Mary de Gonzaga, her eyes shut, lying straight on her back, she seemed a beautiful picture of death. A few hours after she was up again, serving any who needed it.'

On 3 November 'we rose at about daybreak and found ourselves near the entrance of the Dardanelles. Miss Nightingale was on deck looking very worn.' Eventually 'we thankfully landed at Scutari . . . at a rough little pier'.

These poor women, after the ordeal of such a journey, were not welcome when they arrived at the hospital at Scutari. The regulations issued by the Army Medical Department said that

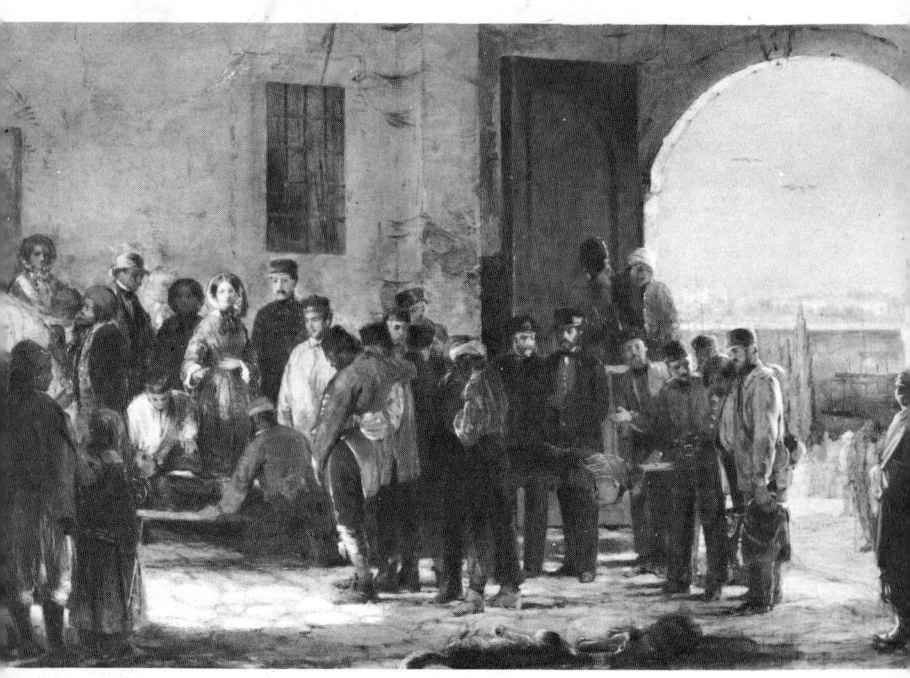

Florence Nightingale receives the wounded at Scutari . . .

female nurses, were 'an unwise indulgence unfavourable to medical discipline and to the recovery of patients'. So the army doctors looked at these intruding women suspiciously.

At first the nurses were not allowed to do anything except prepare dressings and cook food. Only when the casualties poured into the hospital and the doctors were unable to cope were Florence Nightingale and her nurses welcomed in the sick wards.

Sister Margaret Goodman, of the same religious order as Sister Sarah Terrot, describes–or tries to–conditions in the hospital at Scutari:

> 'For about a week after our arrival we were occupied in making shirts, pillows, slings etc., we thought this time very long, but at length we were summoned, and distributed each to one or other of the almost countless rooms of that gigantic hospital, to seam up the beds. A coarse

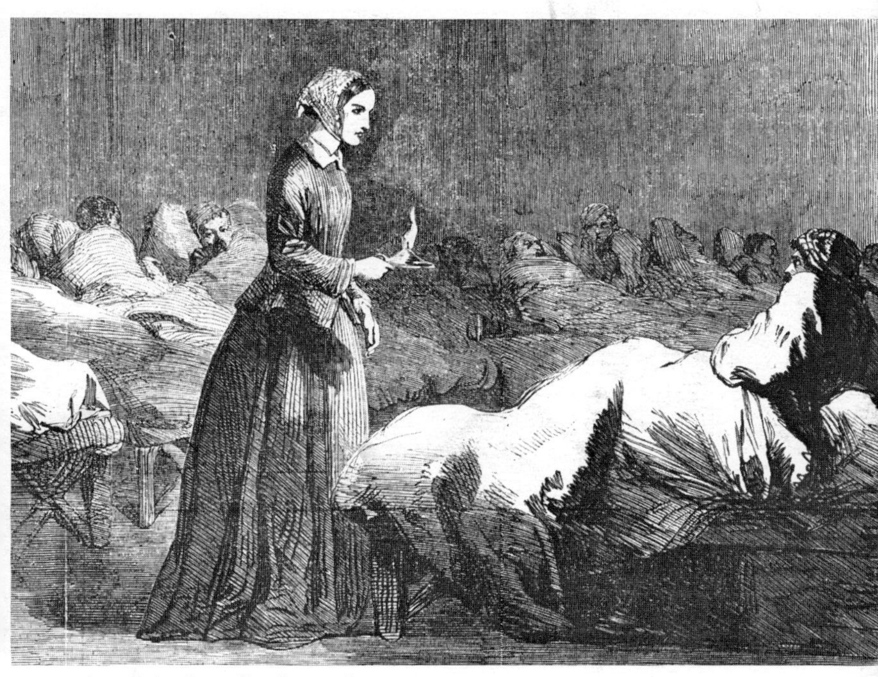
. . . and at night she walks the wards

wrapper, sewn up like a sack on three sides, was hastily filled with chopped straw; our work was to sew the fourth seam, and thus complete the *pallet*. The beds were then laid on the floor about a foot apart, the line extending round the apartment and leaving a small space in the middle. As we laboured, the wounded were arriving. . . .

'The scene baffles description: horror upon horror crowds upon my mind . . . the misery of the dying was also aggravated by the vermin. . . . Night is specially trying to the sick and wretched, and then on all sides arose the moan of pain or the murmur of *delirium*. At this period there were no night nurses, but Miss Nightingale, lamp in hand, each night traversed alone the four miles of beds. How many lives this lady has been the means of saving . . . is fully known only to herself and to the Unseen who watches our steps. She was peculiarly skilled in the art of soothing;

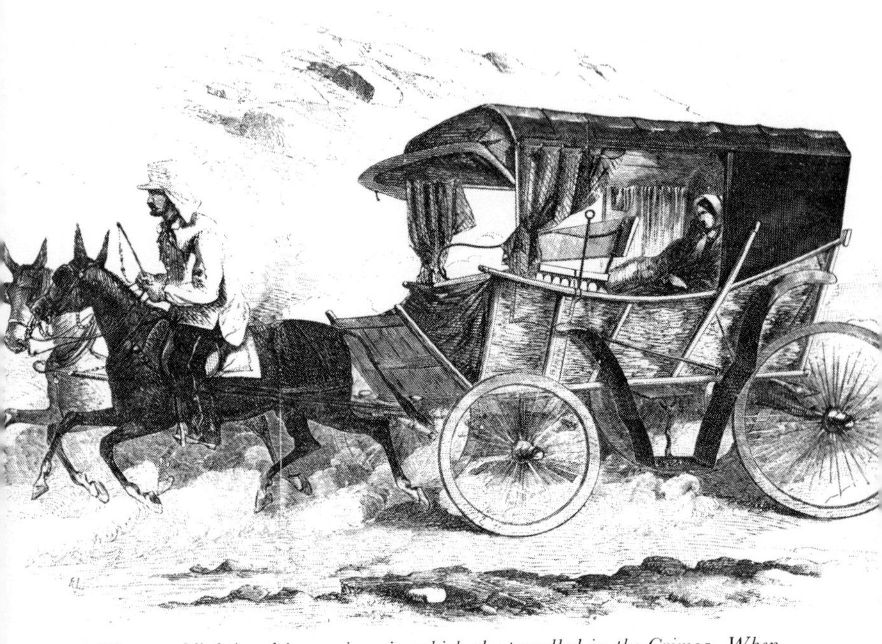

Florence Nightingale's carriage in which she travelled in the Crimea. When visiting the hut hospitals up in the hills she rode on horseback

her gentle sympathising voice and manner always appeared to refresh the sufferer. . . .

'I fear that I should scarcely be credited were I to attempt to describe in detail the noble manner in which the army behaved. They were thankful for the slightest attention, and frequently did all in their power to conceal the pains they endured, lest we should be distressed.'

In 1856 the Russian bid for power was halted and the war ended. So did the picture of a nurse as a useless, untidy creature. Under Florence Nightingale's leadership nurses, for the most part untrained, had done wonderful work under dreadful conditions in the Crimean War. This was recognised by people at home. How much more useful a nurse could be if she was properly trained! Florence Nightingale realised this, and did something about it. In the next chapter we shall see what she achieved.

3 *The Trained Nurse*

'Every woman, or at least almost every woman in England has, at one time or another of her life, charge of the personal health of somebody, whether child or invalid, in other words, every woman is a nurse. It is recognised as the knowledge which every one ought to have–distinct from medical knowledge which only a profession can have. If then, every woman must, at some time or other of her life, become a nurse i.e. have charge of somebody's health, how immense and how valuable would be the produce of her united experience if every woman would think how to nurse. I do not pretend to teach her how, I ask her to teach herself, and for this purpose I venture to give her some hints.'

This is from the Preface of a book 'Notes on Nursing' written by Florence Nightingale for the ordinary woman. It was basic, thorough and dealt with nursing in its widest sense. The content of the book, commonplace enough today, was unheard of in 1859 when it was published. It had a very big sale. Thousands of copies were distributed in factories, villages and schools, and it was translated into French, German and Italian.

After her experiences in the Crimea Florence Nightingale was well aware of the scarcity of reliable nurses and she set her mind to bring about nursing reforms. Although there were training establishments for nurses, she wanted women to be trained as nurses irrespective of their religion or social standing. Her school would send nurses out to teach others. The money was available. People from all over the world had con-

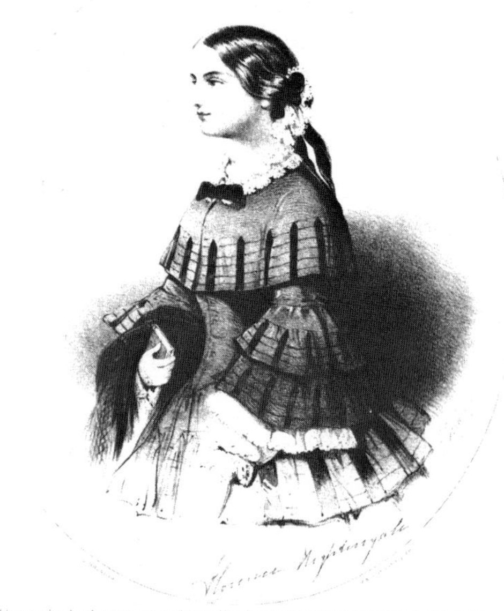

Part of a broadsheet celebrating Florence Nightingale's return from the Crimea. Underneath her picture is quoted an extract from a soldier's letter: '. . . the comfort it was to see even Florence pass, she would speak to one and another, and nod and smile to many more, but she couldn't do it to all, you know, for we lay there by hundreds, but we could kiss her shadow as it fell, and lay our heads on the pillow again content!'

tributed to the Nightingale Fund as a token of appreciation for the work she had done in the Crimean War. The Fund amounted to nearly £50,000 of which almost £10,000 had been contributed by British soldiers.

In the summer of 1860 The Nightingale School for Nurses opened. It was situated on the upper floor of a wing of St Thomas's Hospital in London. There was a separate cubicle for each pupil (or *probationer* as she was called) and Miss Nightingale had personally supervised the decoration which was cheerful and welcoming. There were flowers, books and pictures. All this contrasted with the somewhat grim and dismal surroundings of the hospital.

There were fifteen probationers to begin with. They were required to be 'Sober, Honest, Truthful, Trustworthy, Punctual, Quiet and Orderly, Cleanly and Neat'. They were expected to become (amongst other things) skilful 'in the dressing of blisters, burns, sores, wounds, and in applying *fomentations*, *poultices* and minor dressings. In the application of *leeches*, externally and internally. In the management of helpless Patients i.e. moving, changing, personal cleanliness of feeding, keeping warm (or cool), preventing and dressing bed sores, managing position of. In making the beds of the Patients, and removal of sheets whilst Patient is in bed. To be competent to cook *gruel*, *arrowroot*, *egg-flip*, puddings, drinks for the sick. To understand *ventilation*. . . . To make strict observations of the sick in the following particulars – the state of secretions, expectoration, pulse, skin, appetite; intelligence as delirium or stupor; breathing, sleep, state of wounds, eruptions, formation of matter, effect of diet or stimulants, and of medicines. And to learn the management of convalescents.'

They were also required to attend operations. Mrs Wardroper, Matron of St Thomas's and Superintendent of the School for twenty-seven years wrote to Miss Nightingale that she had given the original fifteen probationers: '1 *alpaca* dress and *mantle*, 2 print ditto, 3 aprons, 3 collars, 3 caps, 1 Bonnet, 1 pair galoshes. I have now a winter dress to provide, but I shall not exceed £4.'

There had been opposition to the school – mainly from men. A doctor, writing before the school was opened commented, 'we always engage the nurses without any character, as no respectable person would undertake so disagreeable an office'. Mr John F. South, a senior surgeon at St Thomas's Hospital considered nurses were 'in much the same position as housemaids and require little teaching beyond that of poultice-making which is easily acquired, the enforcement of cleanliness and attention to the patient's wants'. When it was proposed that a training school should be established in the very hospital at which he was senior surgeon he exploded, 'We have within our own hospitals all the appliances for making the best sisters . . . a training institution for our sisters or nurses is entirely unneeded and *superfluous*.'

Miss Nightingale brushed such opposition aside. It was a minor obstacle compared with what she had had to fight for in the Crimea. She kept a close watch on the School. Reports were sent to her of the progress made by each probationer. She gave instructions that each one was to visit her at her home–away from the hospital–so that she could sum them up. She wrote to Mrs Wardroper, 'beginning at the most junior probationers and so work up until I have seen them all–you sending me one every day at 4.0 and sending me her papers the day before.'

The 'papers' recorded the probationer's progress. It is not difficult to imagine the feelings of a probationer, standing alone in front of the formidable Miss Nightingale, in strange surroundings. She would see, in front of Miss Nightingale, the 'papers'. Miss Nightingale would ask questions and from the answers she would know not only how the young woman's training was progressing, but also how satisfactory–or unsatisfactory–the teaching was. At the end of the meeting the probationer would be sent away and Miss Nightingale would make her comments in handwriting.

> 'Miss W. Tittupy, flippant, pretension-y, ambitious, clever, not much feeling; adventurous, underbred, no religion, thought not small beer of herself–proficiency in wards does not justify this.
>
> 'Miss B. As poor a two-fisted thing as ever I saw. No love of the thing. No heart in it. Wants amusement. Has plenty of time in afternoon for Diaries and Cases but wants to go out and do needlework.
>
> 'Nurse E. Gets up early to mis-inform herself: terrible gossip, flighty, flirty, not thorough: no use.
>
> 'Miss H. If there is anything in her, it requires a hand pump to get it out.
>
> 'Nurse F. As self-comfortable but kindly a Jack-ass (or Joan-ass) as ever I saw. Thinks she does everything well.'

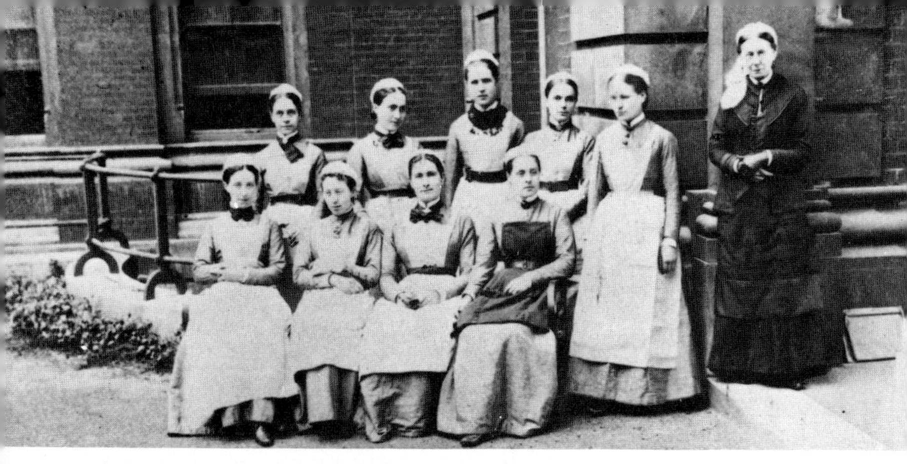

Above: *Mrs Wardroper (in black), superintendent of the Nightingale School for Nurses outside St Thomas's Hospital with some of the probationers*

Nurse Rutherford — March 25/24 /73

Came March 6/72

{7 wks: Medical Female
Miss Parkinson

3 wks: Medical Male: Bull

{4 months: Surgical Male
Miss Cameron {Leopold & Edward

1 mo: S.M. Albert
Miss Pringle

1 wk: S.M. Leopold Miss Airy

{7 wks: back to Albert
Miss Pringle

{9 wks: Surgical Female
Elizabeth Miss Hawthorn

now on Staff night duty
in Leopold: S.M. Miss Airy

Miss Cameron
...ight the most
fortnight on night duty
night duty (special

most capital little woman
no education but one can't find
it in one's heart to regret it
seems as good as she can be
but regrets want of education
not conceited. No complaints
an enthusiasm for her work
for her Sisters

Left: *pencil comments in Florence Nightingale's handwriting on one of the probationers who came to her to report progress. The general comment at the foot is worth deciphering*

And yet, 'Miss G. came a deal too smart [in appearance] but is so nice, unaffected and joyous' was as common as the critical comment.

Rebecca Strong entered the School in June 1867 at the age of twenty-four (she died in 1944, over a hundred years old). She recollects what it was like:

> 'Each pupil had a cubicle in which to sleep, and there was a common dining-room with a neatly appointed table. Very little was expected from us as progress was slow in regard to organised teaching. Kindness, watchfulness, cleanliness and guarding against bedsores were well *ingrained.* A few stray lectures were given, one I remember especially, I think it was on the Chemistry of Life or some such title; it caused me to get a book on the subject which I found most useful. There was a dummy on which to practise bandaging . . . also a skeleton and some ancient medical books, one fortunately on *Anatomy* for those who attempted self-education. . . . I must say that although Florence Nightingale had scrubbed floors and cleaned brasses at Kaiserswerth, she did not ask this of her pupils, the whole time on duty was given to the patients. The directions on medicine bottles were given in Latin, therefore some Latin *abbreviations* had to be learned, which was not difficult. . . . Temperature taking and chart keeping were medical student's work. I was once asked by a surgeon to take a temperature and, on being found by the sister in the act, was severely reprimanded for doing the student's work, but from that time it gradually became the work of a nurse.
>
> 'On Saturday mornings two pupils were told off to make cakes for Sunday. Outdoor uniform was provided as well as in; the outdoor consisting of a shawl and bonnet worn over one's ordinary dress. A pupil was told off now and again to trim the bonnets: I had my turn so you see we were supposed to be useful in various ways. A pupil, or probationer as she was called, on entering the Nightingale School signed on for [three] years, but it did not follow

that she remained in St Thomas's for that time. After one year's residence there she was supposed to have gained sufficient knowledge to become a pioneer in other hospitals, at home and abroad.'

It was from the School that nurses were sent all over the world to train others. A Report on the School issued in 1897 tells us that from 'the opening of the School in 1860 to the end of 1897 a total of 1,452 Candidates have been admitted and 864 have, after completing a year's training, received appointments in St Thomas's or some other approved public Hospital or Infirmary, or District Nursing Institute for the benefit of the sick poor'. It might be thought that over a period of thirty-seven years, the 'wastage' was on the high side. This could be accounted for by probationers getting married and also by the high standard Miss Nightingale set, for she believed in quality, not quantity.

Florence Nightingale had proved to the men that nurses needed training but the Nightingale School could not teach every probationer. Some received excellent teaching – mostly from the London hospitals – but at lesser establishments it was not so thorough and occasionally probationers were used as cheap labour. How skilled, then, was a 'trained' nurse? It depended where she had received her training and that was not a satisfactory situation. In 1886 a proposal was made that every nurse should be officially recognised as trained provided she passed an examination, when her name would be placed on a register. Only nurses on the register would be considered 'trained'.

Florence Nightingale objected. The nurse 'may have gone through a first-rate course, plenty of examinations, and we may find nothing inside', she said. 'It may be the difference between a Nurse nursing and a Nurse reading a book on Nursing. Unless it bear fruit, it is all gilding and *veneering*. No Nurse can stand still. She must go forward or she will go backward every year. We grow down, if we don't grow up, every year.'

Despite such comments from so important a person, the

British Nurses Association was formed to press for a register of nurses. Miss Nightingale, now seventy years of age, fought against the scheme, not so much because she objected to the register, but because the time was not yet ripe for it, and she mistrusted examinations. She believed in practical experience and thought the nurses would be worse if they did examinations instead of concentrating on nursing. Probationers could become excellent nurses but might be stupid at passing examinations. On the other hand there would be those who shone at examinations but were not necessarily good nurses by Miss Nightingale's standards.

It was to be a long drawn-out battle. Despite her age Miss Nightingale was not the sort of woman to give in. Ranged against her was a younger generation – hardly less formidable than herself – and the doctors drawn into the fight took sides 'for' and 'against' registration. There were mass meetings and legal arguments in the courts.

The case for registration gained strength because registers had been set up for other professions such as doctors in 1858 and school teachers were seeking registration too. The Midwives Act of 1902 was to introduce a register for midwives. In 1903 a Bill for the registration of nurses was laid before Parliament but rejected. A Select Committee was instead appointed to look into the matter. The Committee found in favour of registration and suggested how it should be done. In 1904 another Nurses' Registration Bill was placed before Parliament. Members of Parliament were besieged by constituents pleading 'for' or 'against' the bill. There was great activity in both camps and despite the demand for registration there were many influential people against it. The Government were cautious. It was difficult to find time for the Bill, they said – or that was the excuse.

Every year from 1904 to 1914 the Bill got no further in Parliament, and when in 1914 the First World War broke out, the Bill was dropped. There were other more pressing matters. It was, however, due to the war that the Government realised how useful a register would have been. As the war went on,

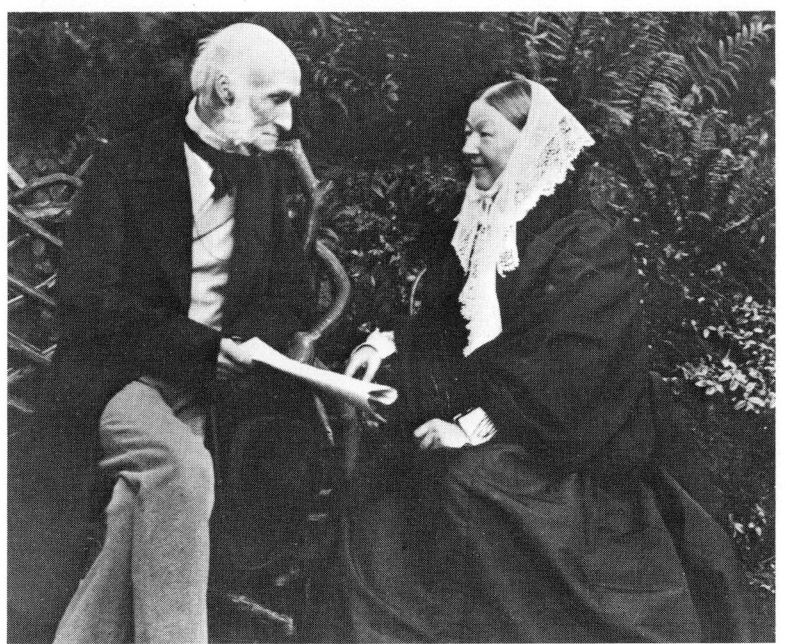

Florence Nightingale in her old age, with her brother-in-law, Sir Harry Verney, Bart. at Claydon House, Buckinghamshire, 1889. Sir Harry married Parthenope who died a year later

year after year, and the appalling casualties crowded the hospitals, the demand for nurses was acute. If there had been a register, how easy it would have been to find trained nurses!

In 1919, a year after the war was over (Florence Nightingale had been dead nine years) the Nurses Registration Act was passed by Parliament. To become a registered nurse you had to be twenty-one years old and have had training for three (in some cases four) years at a recognised training school. There was a preliminary examination after one year's training and a final examination on subjects connected with the branch of nursing you wanted to take up.

Over the years the examinations and training have changed to keep step with modern medicine, but the Register still exists and those on it may add S.R.N. after their name to show they are State Registered Nurses.

4 Barber-surgeons, Physicians and a Student's Diary

Outside some barbers shops you sometimes see a blue and white pole – the barber's pole. In the sixteenth century the barber was also a surgeon and the patient was given a stick or pole to hold on to during the operation. Gripping the pole helped to lessen the pain because at that time there were no anaesthetics and no pain-killing drugs. When the pole wasn't in use it was hung outside the shop as a sign. The blue stripe on the pole is a symbol of the blue veins from which blood flowed; the white stripe represents bandages.

From 1540 until 1745 London barbers who wanted to practise surgery had to be licensed by the United Company of Barbers and Surgeons. The Company gave good instruction at the Barber-Surgeons' Hall in the City of London. Samuel Pepys in 1663 attended some lectures there. First he dined with the doctors in the Hall. The meal was magnificent, he records in his Diary, and afterwards he went with his hosts to see a body 'which was a lusty fellow, a seaman that was hanged for robbery. I did touch the dead body with my bare hand; it felt cold, but methought it was a very unpleasant sight.' Later 'we went into a private room where I perceive they prepare the bodies. Thence with great satisfaction back to the Company, where I heard good discourse, and so to the afternoon lecture upon the heart and lungs etc.'

In the eighteenth century there was already a difference between medicine and surgery. The physician had generally been to a university and was probably a fellow of the Royal College of Physicians that had been formed in 1518 by

 Henry VIII. The purpose of the College was to protect people

'*Shaving, bleeding and teeth drawn with a touch*', states the sign outside the Barber-Surgeon's house. You can see him at work through the window. In the Street there is chaos. You can almost hear the noise, feel the heat of the fire, and smell the contents of that chamber-pot cascading on to the luckless watchman below. Entitled 'Night' this picture was 'invented, painted, engraved and published' in 1738 by William Hogarth (1697–1764)

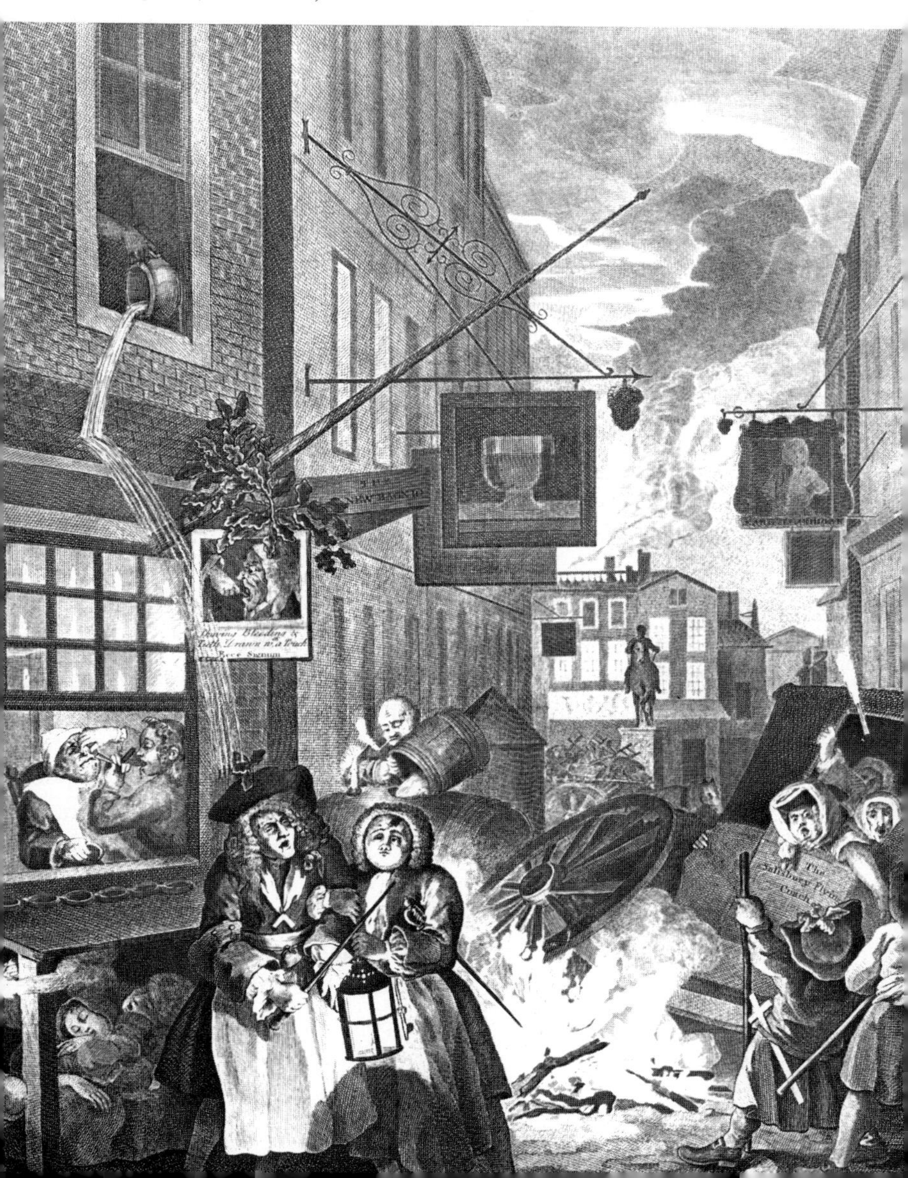

against bad doctors, or, as its charter said, 'to curb the *audacity* of those wicked men who shall profess medicine more for the sake of their *avarice* than from the assurance of any good conscience'. In 1667 the Royal College of Physicians of Ireland was established, and of Scotland in 1681.

The surgeon was not so well educated as the physician and was of a lower social standing. Only when the surgeon separated from the barber did he achieve recognition in the medical world. It was due to the influence of pioneers such as William Hunter (1718–83) who, in 1743 advertised lectures on surgery to which 'would be added . . . the application of bandages'. From such beginnings Hunter and others by their teaching improved the surgeon's knowledge. Finally the surgeons were brought together in a society through which teaching could be done. Consequently the surgeon became a member of the Royal College of Surgeons of Edinburgh (1778), or of Ireland (1784) or of London (1800).

After the surgeon came the *apothecary* – a Freeman of the Society of Apothecaries in London – who actually attended the patient (provided he could pay!). After seeing the patient the apothecary would go to a coffee house to see the physician he generally consulted. The apothecary would describe the patient's ills and the physician wrote out a prescription in Latin with instructions as to how the patient was to be treated. The apothecary returned to the patient, carried out the physician's instructions and called a barber-surgeon if any bleeding was required. The physician only saw the patient who was seriously ill.

Lastly came the unlicensed 'doctor' who treated the poor and destitute in their own homes. Often they were kind men with limited knowledge who did the best they could for their patients.

There were also 'quacks' – men (and women) without any training, who stood in the market place and claimed to be able to cure every kind of ill – at a price. They talked well and convincingly, and people who had given up hope of being restored to health paid their money for the 'cures' that were offered. No doubt in some cases, the 'cure' worked merely because the patient had faith in the treatment, or because the treatment received did no harm and the complaint cured itself. But many people were bitterly disappointed.

In the eighteenth century the training of doctors and surgeons developed still further through medical schools and attendance at voluntary general hospitals where medical students 'walked' the wards and learnt at first hand about the ills and diseases they would have to cope with when their training was finished. Such hospitals as the Westminster, Guy's and St George's in London, The Royal Infirmary in Edinburgh, Leeds Infirmary, Birmingham General Hospital – all founded in the eighteenth century – became training hospitals for the students.

We have seen in the previous chapter the reasons that led to the registration of nurses. Can you see why it was just as important that there should be a 'register' of those practising medicine? It was essential that there should be standards of training and education and that only those who had gained diplomas or degrees should be considered qualified. In 1858 the Medical Act ensured there was a 'single register' for all medical practitioners – doctors, consultants, surgeons. The Act was administered by what is now the General Medical Council. The full Council consists of 47 members, some of whom are appointed by the Government, others by learned medical societies, and by election by the rank and file of medical men. The Council disciplines the doctors etc., on the register. If a doctor or surgeon on the register seriously breaks the law, or breaks the rules of the medical professional (such as advertising, 'poaching' another doctor's patients) he can be made to appear before the Council. His misbehaviour may be so serious that it amounts to 'infamous professional conduct' and the Council strikes the doctor's name off the register. When this happens the doctor can no longer practise medicine; his livelihood has been taken away from him. After a period of time he can apply to the Council to be restored to the register and very often he is given another chance.

In 1860–two years after the Medical Act–a student, Shepherd Taylor–left his Norfolk home to come to London. He wanted to become a doctor, and during his four years of study kept a diary. On 29 September 1860 he left home in the morning 'taking up my residence at Dyer's Buildings, Holborn, a sort of courtyard or *cul-de-sac* leading out of Holborn, in the vicinity of Gray's Inn Road. Mrs May, my future landlady, a homely, good tempered looking body, gave me a *cordial* reception. Dyer's Buildings is rather a dull gloomy place to live in, but free from the noise and turmoil of the main *thoroughfare*, an advantage not to be despised by one engaged in studious occupation.' (Dyer's Buildings faces the Prudential Assurance in Holborn. Up to 1973 it cannot have changed much since Taylor's student days, but his 'rooms' became offiices. Now, alas, the *cul-de-sac* is being 'developed'. It is unlikely to remain 'dull and gloomy', and it certainly no longer escapes 'the noise and turmoil of the main thoroughfare').

On 1 October Taylor 'paid a visit to King's College, Somerset House, in the morning. The sub-dean who had to put his signature to my matriculation card, appeared to be a very *genial* sort of gentleman. . . . In the evening I commenced my career of *dissipation* by going to the Strand Theatre, where we had three or four very lively comedies, which pleased me not a little.'

The Medical Department of King's College was established in 1831, but it was not until 1840 that the first King's College Hospital was opened close to Lincoln's Inn Fields. It was in the hospital that the students had an opportunity of seeing what they had learnt at the College put to practical use. Students were expected to be 'regular in their attendance at Divine Worship in the College Chapel, particularly on Sundays in the *forenoon*' and up to 1913 a rule existed–but not obeyed–'that *post-mortems* must not be performed at such times as would interfere with the presence of the hospital porters at Divine Service in the Chapel'.

Taylor's diary gives an interesting picture of a medical student's life in mid-Victorian England. In many ways it follows the pattern of a medical student's life today. He criticises and makes fun of the learned professors who taught him, he makes 'sick' jokes about cutting up bodies and investigating parts of the human anatomy, he suffers at examination time like the best of us:

'11th October 1860. I purchased a skeleton for £2, and for £1 1*s* a skull sawn through horizontally and vertically..

1st November 1860. Written examination in Chemistry, in which I acquitted myself indifferently, chiefly from having a bad pen.

9th November 1860. Had my silver watch stolen by a rascally thief as I was watching the Lord Mayor's procession in Fleet Street. I positively saw the wretch snatch it away from my pocket, but he passed it on so quickly to an *accomplice* that I felt it a hopeless business to get it back again.

January 7th 1861. Commenced dissecting a leg. Went to a concert in the evening.

January 13th 1861. Fog from the Thames so intense that we were obliged to give up dissecting, being unable to see.

March 1st 1861. Funds getting very low, only 5*s* 9*d* in hand, with a fortnight's rent to pay. Economy must be the order of the day.

March 11th 1861. Examination. . . . Answered the various questions tolerably well, what with my actual knowledge of the subject and *ingenious* guesses, where my knowledge was at fault.

October 8th 1862. Registered my name at the College of Surgeons. Mr Stone, the Registrar or Secretary, not particularly civil, recommending me to be quicker in my answers, whereupon I gave them as short and sharp as possible, which I could plainly see had the desired effect of teaching Mr Stone that I was not a man to be set upon.'

It is when one comes upon an entry like this that it is difficult to believe it took place a little over a hundred years ago and not in the middle ages:

'October 20th 1862. Saw Mrs Catherine Wilson, a nurse, hanged at the Old Bailey for poisoning her friend, Mrs Soames, seven years ago. It was certainly a very *gruesome spectacle*. Mrs C. W. however, behaved very coolly, and being a stoutish woman "fell beautiful", to use the words of an illiterate bystander.'

Taylor attended a number of hangings as part of the crowd. This entry is revealing:

'March 7th 1863. The Princess Alexandra [wife of Edward, Prince of Wales–the future Edward VII] was expected to make her public entry in London via the Strand and Temple Bar today. As ill-luck would have it, at 4.30 a.m. I had to attend a mid-wifery case in a courtyard leading out of the Strand close to Temple Bar. As the case was rather a slow and *tedious* one, I was able to take my stand in the street, where I should have an excellent view of the Prince and Princess; but at 3 p.m. just as the Royal procession was almost in sight and the drums began to beat, my services were required by the patient. However, the good lady, thinking she could hold out a trifle longer, I returned to the street and had a fair view after all.'

More grimly:

'March 20th 1863. Attended out-patient department, 120 patients old and new. Dreadfully tedious and uninteresting work. About two minutes bestowed on each case, a pure farce in fact.

May 4th 1863. Midwifery case at 12 night. Wife of a stableman to a cab proprietor, the room saturated with the odour of ammonia from the stalls directly underneath it. One of the horses got loose during the night and kicked about him with such energy that we had to go below and fasten him up again.'

It was part of his medical education at that time to observe:

 'June 5th 1863. The physicians attached to English hospitals receive no [pay] for their services at the hospitals. Their work is purely voluntary. They get their living from their patients outside the hospital, who naturally receive the lion's share of their attention. Three or four times a week they make a hurried round in the hospital wards and then go forth to earn golden guineas outside.'

Shepherd Taylor qualified the next year and returned to his native Norfolk.

5 *Petticoat Physician*

Today there are about 14,000 registered women doctors. In 1859 there was one. Here is the story of one woman's struggle to become a doctor.

She was born Elizabeth Garrett in 1836. First the family lived in London, but when Elizabeth was four years old they went to live at Aldeburgh in Suffolk, making the journey from London by sea. Her father, Newson Garrett, was not a rich man until he lived at Aldeburgh. There he worked hard and by 1850 he had become wealthy with numerous business interests in the neighbourhood. He built a mansion, Alde House, surrounded by gardens and paddocks. In such happy surroundings Elizabeth grew up with five sisters and four brothers.

When she was eighteen she went to stay with some friends in the north, at Gateshead. There she met a young woman, some six years her senior, by the name of Emily Davies, daughter of the Rector of Gateshead. Emily was amusing and impatient. She protested against the patronising attitude towards young women of her generation who, it was assumed, were incapable of following any worthwhile career and consequently were not worth educating. In those days the woman's place was in the home looking after ageing parents, eventually marrying and bearing numerous children. Emily had great influence on Elizabeth and they became firm friends. Emily's (at that time) revolutionary ideas fired Elizabeth to do something worthwhile with her life. But what?

As the eldest unmarried daughter in a large household she should have been busy. There were her brothers and sisters to keep an eye on, the garden to tend, stables, glasshouses, piggeries–all the trappings of a wealthy home needed her attention. But it was not enough. She was restless. Her hands might be busy, but her mind was not. Later in life she remembered, 'I was a young woman living at home with nothing to do in what authors call "comfortable circumstances". But I was wicked enough not to be comfortable. I was full of energy and

Elizabeth Garrett Anderson in middle age

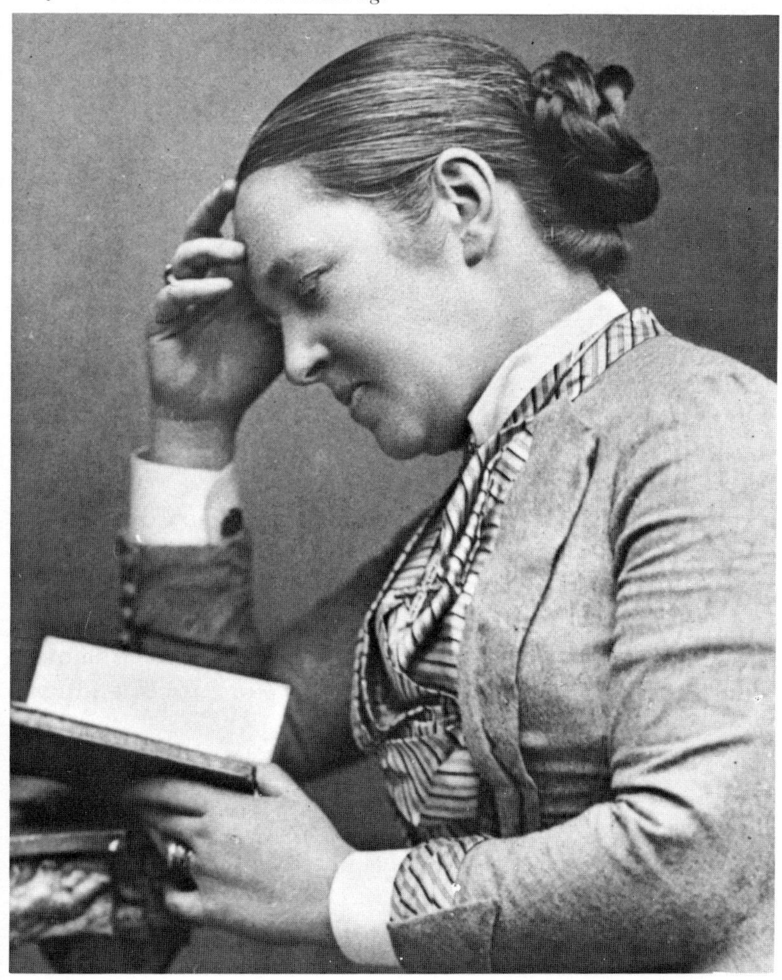

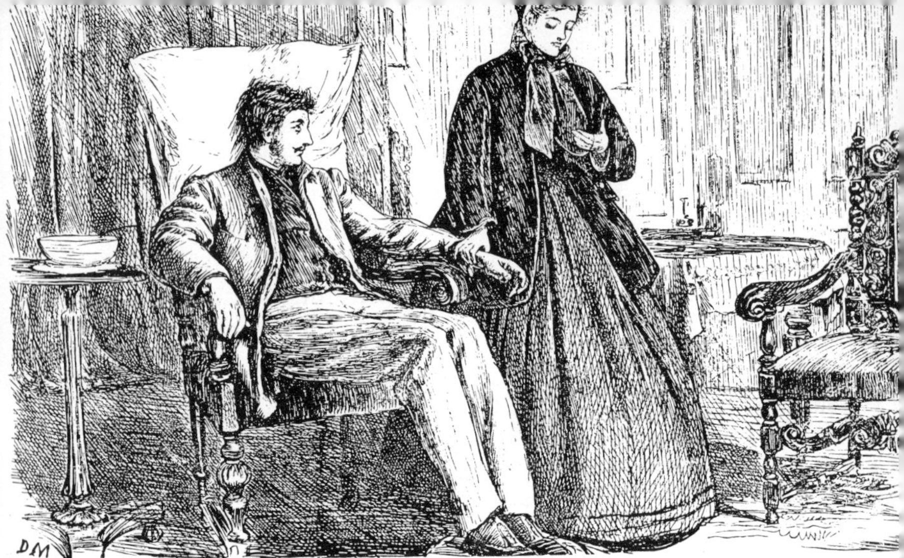

LADY PHYSICIANS

WHO IS THIS INTERESTING INVALID? IT IS YOUNG REGINALD DE BRACES, WHO HAS SUCCEEDED IN CATCHING A BAD COLD IN ORDER THAT HE MIGHT SEND FOR THAT RISING PRACTITIONER, DR. ARABELLA BOLUS!

The invalid is obviously love-sick! Punch *makes fun of the woman doctor*

vigour and of the discontent which goes with unemployed activities. Everything seemed wrong to me.'

These words seem to echo those spoken by Florence Nightingale. Elizabeth and Florence came from different backgrounds but they shared the same discontent. Elizabeth's education was not impressive. She was taught by a governess until she was thirteen and then went to the Boarding School for Ladies at 4 Dartmouth Road, London, S.E., near Blackheath to be 'finished'. A short tour abroad, a visit to the Great Exhibition of 1851 and she was considered ready to face the world. But Elizabeth was searching for a meaning to her life. There was no 'call from God' such as Florence Nightingale had experienced.

It was after she had heard a lecture by Dr Elizabeth Blackwell that she whispered to her young sister, 'I'm going to be a doctor'. Little did she know what was in store for her. Dr Blackwell, an Englishwoman, had graduated in medicine abroad and had come to England to place her name on the Medical Register. She was the first woman to have achieved it and everyone criticised or laughed at her.

'I'm going to be a doctor,' repeated Elizabeth Garrett to her parents. She wrote to Emily Davies, 'I have just concluded a satisfactory talk with Father on the medical subject. He was not at all disposed to oppose me actively. He does not like it, I think.' But later she reported to Emily another conversation with father. 'He said the whole idea was disgusting that he could not *entertain* it for a moment. I asked what there was to make doctoring more disgusting than nursing, which women were also doing, and which ladies had done publicly in the Crimea. He could not tell me. . . . I think he will probably come round in time. I mean to renew the subject pretty often.'

Secretly she arranged with the schoolmaster at Aldeburgh to coach her in Greek and Latin. Her mother was so upset that she retired to bed and made herself ill through crying. 'You will kill your mother if you go on,' Elizabeth was warned. Elizabeth did not heed the warning. She did not believe her mother would die, and she was right. Her mother lived to be ninety.

She was also right about her father. He did 'come round in time', slowly but surely. In 1860 we see father and daughter in Harley Street calling on the leading medical consultants and asking how a woman could become a doctor. The reception they got was not encouraging. Some were polite, some were rude, others smirked, none offered any advice. The more obstacles they met, the more Mr Garrett rallied to his daughter's cause. So much so that later he wrote to her, 'I have resolved in my own mind after deep and painful consideration not to oppose your wishes and views, and so far as expense is involved, I will do all I can in justice to my other children to assist you in your study. Your dear mother is very anxious.' He was as good as his word and in the future battles to be fought he was a tower of strength.

Elizabeth confided in her father at every stage. She also consulted her ally Emily Davies. Elizabeth reported every move; Emily was full of advice, rallying to her cause, and stiffening Elizabeth when she wilted, like a whalebone in a corset.

How to make a beginning? Elizabeth wondered. She turned to a good teaching hospital – the Middlesex in London. Being female she was not permitted to enter as a medical student, but she was acceptable as a nurse. She was put to work in a surgical ward in the hope that the horrors she would see (this was in the days before anaesthetics) would put her to flight. On the contrary, her interest increased. Although she was a nurse in name, she became more of a student. The staff even offered to coach her privately. From Elizabeth's standpoint it was becoming ridiculous that she shouldn't be accepted as a student. She applied accordingly and was at first refused. She persisted and the authorities accepted her for some special lectures. She was triumphant. 'I have had to sign my name in the College books in token that I will not smoke, but will in every way *comport* myself as a gentleman.'

She sat examinations and received a Certificate of Honour in each subject. A friendly examiner implored her to keep the news of her success from the male students! Then the blow fell. One day, a visiting physician asked the class a question which none of the male students could answer. Only Elizabeth knew the answer. The infuriated male students demanded that she should be dismissed, and Elizabeth was told that she would not be permitted to attend any more lectures other than those she had paid for.

There she was, then, back at the beginning having gained experience but no further on the way to becoming a doctor. She discovered another door open to her. The Hall of Apothecaries permitted women to sit for their examinations provided they had served an apprenticeship for five years with a qualified doctor. Elizabeth found a doctor who would instruct her and she prepared to take the examination in 1866. If she passed she would be a Licentiate of the Society of Apothecaries which would enable her name to be placed on the Medical Register, but – to Elizabeth – it was an unsatisfactory qualification. She would not be able to work in a hospital, for example. The only worthwhile qualification was to become an M.D. –

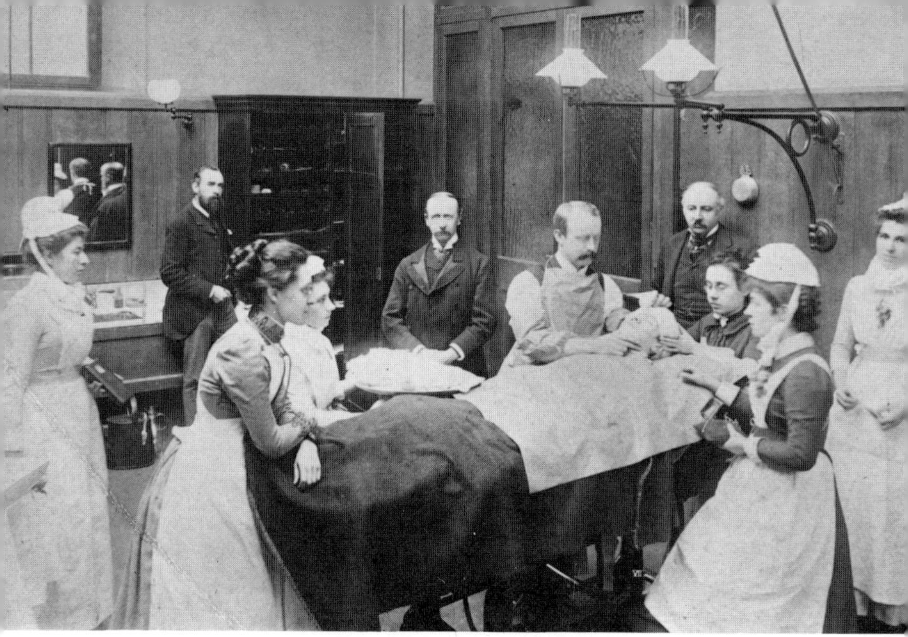

Women students in an operating theatre at the then London School of Medicine for Women about 1890, later to become the Royal Free Hospital School of Medicine

Doctor of Medicine. She would then be on equal terms with the men in the profession.

She then battled with the University of London for permission to take the matriculation examination – an essential step before entry was granted to study at a university. She was refused permission. Her father took legal advice. Letters were written by and to influential people, but without any success. It was not until 1877 that London University opened its doors to women.

She next turned her attention to Edinburgh University. She applied for permission to take the matriculation examination and she actually received from the Secretary of the University a ticket permitting her to do so. Furthermore, to her amazement, she was allowed to take tickets for other subjects. Triumphantly she held tickets in her hand, not only for matriculation but for the anatomy lectures as well. This was unbelievable! Indeed it was. The Heads of the University met and decided that the matriculation and anatomy class tickets had been given without proper authority. She was ordered to give them back and that, as far as the authorities were concerned, was that. But they had not reckoned with Elizabeth and her father. Once again legal advice was taken. More letters were written; outcries at the injustice of it all fell on deaf ears, but there was no hope of her being examined there.

A less courageous person might have given in, but by 1865 she was now able to take the examination at the Hall of the Apothecaries, as she had served her apprenticeship. Even the Apothecaries tried to go back on their word of four years earlier by saying that women were not permitted to sit the examinations. Mr Garrett consulted lawyers and this time he won. Elizabeth was permitted to sit for the examination, although the Apothecaries altered the regulations so that future candidates must have worked in a recognised medical school (from which women were excluded). She passed the examination with flying colours but 'no doubt', commented a writer in the medical journal 'The Lancet' of 7 October 1865, 'the examiners had due regard to her sex and omitted all those subjects of examination which would be shocking to the female mind.'

As soon as she was qualified Mr Garrett leased a house for his daughter at 20 Upper Berkeley Street in London, near Marble Arch. What should she put on the brassplate? 'I don't like "Miss Garrett" on the door,' she wrote. 'It is only like a dressmaker. Louie [a sister] strongly advises "Elizabeth Garrett, L.S.A." [Licentiate of the Society of Apothecaries] and a night bell.'

With the brass plate outside the door she waited for patients. She was prepared to attend male patients but there was always the possibility of scandal. Her best course, she thought, was to specialise in the treatment of women and children.

In 1865 there was an epidemic of Asiatic Cholera in Egypt which arrived in Britain the following summer. Just as Florence Nightingale's nurses had been welcomed only when the Crimea battle casualties became overwhelming and the men could not cope, so hostility towards Elizabeth as a woman doctor disappeared in the wake of this appalling epidemic. She opened a dispensary at 69 Seymour Place–near her consulting room–and as a result of the work she did there, her reputation grew.

But she was not yet a qualified doctor of medicine and she was determined that she should be. She decided, therefore, to become a Doctor of Medicine in Paris. The Faculty of Medicine there was prepared to accept women. On the other hand Elizabeth did not want to go to France to study. She was too busy at her dispensary. She resigned from committees, gave up going to see friends and devoted what little spare time she had to revision. 'I am giving up all society in order to keep the evenings free for work, as this saves both time and energy,' she wrote. She studied late into the night and rose early before breakfast to study more. In the horse cab that took her on her 'rounds' of patients, she studied in between visits. She was then thirty-two years of age, fighting a lone battle and determined to win. In 1870 she was ready to take the final examination to become a Doctor of Medicine. In June she wrote to a friend, 'My Paris summons came this morning. Drink to my becoming a great physician on the 15th with thirty years of vigour before one; surely this is not too much to look for?'

On 15 June Elizabeth Garrett stood before her examiners at the Paris Faculty of Medicine dressed in the customary long gown of black wool with stitched bands. Her head was uncovered and in her hand she carried her thesis (an essay on a particular medical subject necessary for the examination) from which she read. Questions were fired at her–in French. She emerged triumphant. The correspondent of the medical journal 'The Lancet' reported that 'the hall was literally crowded with students, and, on Miss Garrett's crossing the courtyard to leave the school, I observed with pleasure that almost all the students gallantly bowed'.

Back in England she was acclaimed. Journals hostile to women doctors reluctantly agreed that tributes were due to Elizabeth Garrett, M.D. Universities and hospitals which had cold-shouldered her made clucking noises of approval. Never again would any woman, wishing to become a qualified doctor, have to overcome the obstacles that Elizabeth did. Now she was accepted by the leading (male!) physicians of London. It must have seemed a long time since she and her father walked down Harley Street knocking on the doors for advice!

Now she was urged to serve on important committees and people asked for her opinions on all sorts of problems, not necessarily connected with medicine.

On 9 February 1871 at the age of thirty-five she married James Skelton Anderson who was in the shipping business. They had two sons and a daughter. Elizabeth died in 1917 at the age of eighty-one.

Inspired by Elizabeth Garrett Anderson, other women, equally frustrated at being more or less excluded from a profession dominated by men, started dispensaries or small hospitals where the staff consisted entirely of women. Dr Annie McCall in 1887 broke away from mission work to open a clinic that became the Clapham Maternity Hospital, since renamed the Annie McCall Maternity Hospital in south-west London. The Duchess of York Hospital for Babies was founded in 1914 by Dr Catherine Chisholm as the Manchester Babies Hospital. Dr Sophia Jex-Blake started a small dispensary in Edinburgh in 1878; it is now the Bruntsfield Hospital. Dr Alice McLaren and Dr Elizabeth Pace founded in 1902 what has now become the Redlands Hospital for Women in Glasgow.

But the greatest memorial is, perhaps, the Elizabeth Garrett Anderson Hospital in Euston Road, London. (It was known as the New Hospital for Women until after her death–she would not have it bear her name during her lifetime.) The hospital originated in 1872 above Elizabeth's dispensary in Seymour Place. In 1874 a move was made to larger premises in Marylebone Road. The Euston Road building, specially constructed, opened in 1890 when Euston Road was quiet. Today the building is outdated and the noisy traffic streams past. And if you have time to look at No. 20 Upper Berkeley Street when you visit London you will see a plaque on the

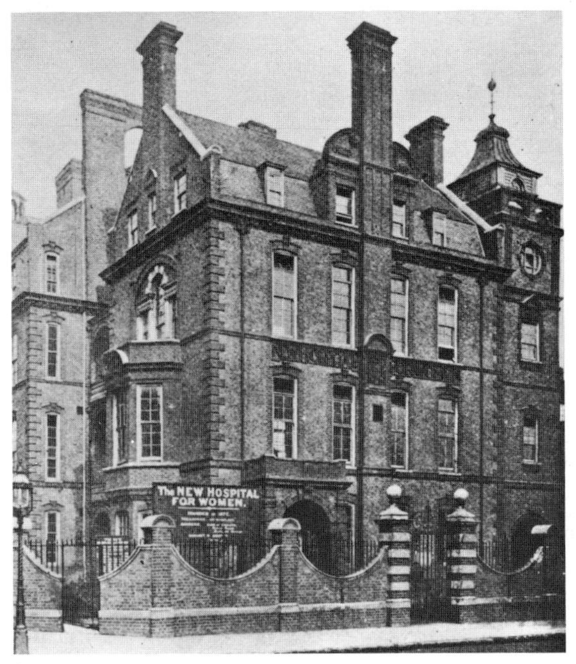

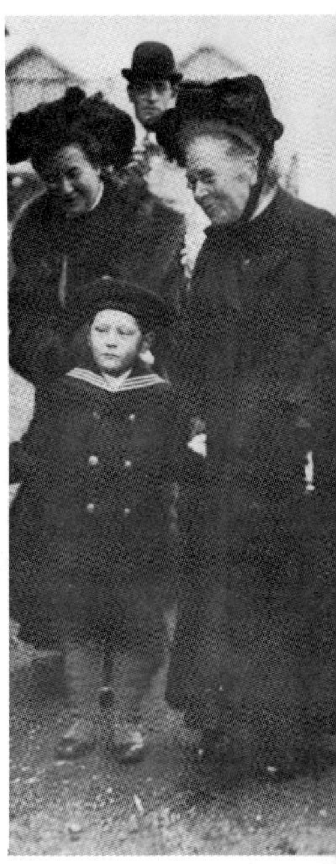

Above left: *The Hospital for Women in Euston Road, London, now the Elizabeth Garrett Anderson Hospital. (She would not have it named after her during her lifetime). Opened in 1890, it was nearly closed in the 1970s for economy reasons but people protested so much that it remained open, an old building past which traffic flows continuously*

Above right: *An historic family photograph. Elizabeth Garrett Anderson can be seen on the right. She was Mayor of Aldeburgh and in her seventies. She holds the hand of her grandson Colin. Bending over him is his aunt Dr Louisa Garrett Anderson. The gentleman in the bowler hat at the back is his father, Sir Alan Anderson. This photograph was taken at the opening of the first model yacht sailing pond at Aldeburgh, the year about 1909*

house which states that Elizabeth Garrett Anderson 'the first woman to qualify as a doctor in Britain lived there'.

As a footnote to this chapter it should be recorded that in 1969–nearly one hundred years after Elizabeth Garrett (as she then was) qualified as a doctor–a woman, for the first time, was appointed physician to a reigning monarch, Queen Elizabeth II.

6 *The Victorian Doctor*

'God and the doctor men adore
When sickness comes, but not before;
When health returns and they are righted
God is forgotten and the doctor slighted'

A DOCTOR'S LAMENT.

A small boy in the middle of the last century, watched doctors arrive at a small Sussex village.

> 'They were always on horseback and dressed as a rule in summer, in dark swallow-tailed coats and brass buttons, light waistcoat and breeches, top boots and spurs, and large white tie and frill. . . . Professional jealousy ran very high and it was reported that meeting in a narrow lane, two neighbouring practitioners literally charged each other because neither would give way to the other.'

At that time there was no Health Service. A doctor had to live by the money he received from his patients. When he became a qualified doctor he could either buy a practice from a doctor who wanted to retire, or he could put up a brass plate outside his house bearing his name and qualifications. It cost money to buy a practice, but the patients were there. If he 'put up his plate' he had to wait for patients to come to him and he might well have some anxious years trying to make ends meet.

A newly qualified doctor, John Bradley, has just purchased a practice from a retiring doctor who is showing John round:

> 'You can see for yourself what this practice is like. Nothing grand about it: but, when all's said and done, it's not such

a bad little show. It's *compact* and easy to run, and the patients are not bad folk when you get to know 'em. . . . You'll find it a great comfort, too, having everything on a cash basis: saves you the bother of book-keeping and the unpleasantness of collecting bad debts'

This is from a book 'Dr Bradley Remembers' by Francis Brett Young, a doctor who knew only too well how important prompt payment by patients was.

Here is a doctor who put his 'plate' up and waited.

'On August 8th, 1868 I put up my plate and waited for patients. A consulting-room in a poor locality . . . connected with a chemist's shop. No rent was asked as [the chemist] got all my prescriptions to dispense, upon the profits of which he found the means to enable him to marry. . . . I attended there for an hour, morning and evening. I only obtained very small fees: 1*s* for a consultation, and 1*s* 6*d* to 2*s* for a visit, and half a guinea for a *confinement*. In a short space of time, I was in receipt of, on an average, a pound a day, which was a welcome addition to the income derived from the gradually, but slowly, increasing number of my better-class patients.'

A doctor who went into partnership with another doctor fared little better:

'My work in the first four years was very hard. I worked Sundays and week-days, night and day, and in the first four years I had only 21 days holiday in all. I could afford no carriage and walked to my patients, mile after mile, all day. Now and then, rather than be seen walking up to a door I would take a shilling hansom, only for the appearance of the thing. My first winter, that of 1890, heralded in the first big epidemics of influenza. I myself was ill with it. I fainted in one lady's room, again in my partner's carriage, and once more in my consulting room. But someone HAD to see the patients and I did not lie up, though I could scarcely stand.'

It was not to be wondered at that a doctor's ambition was to attract the 'better-class' type of patient who could afford to

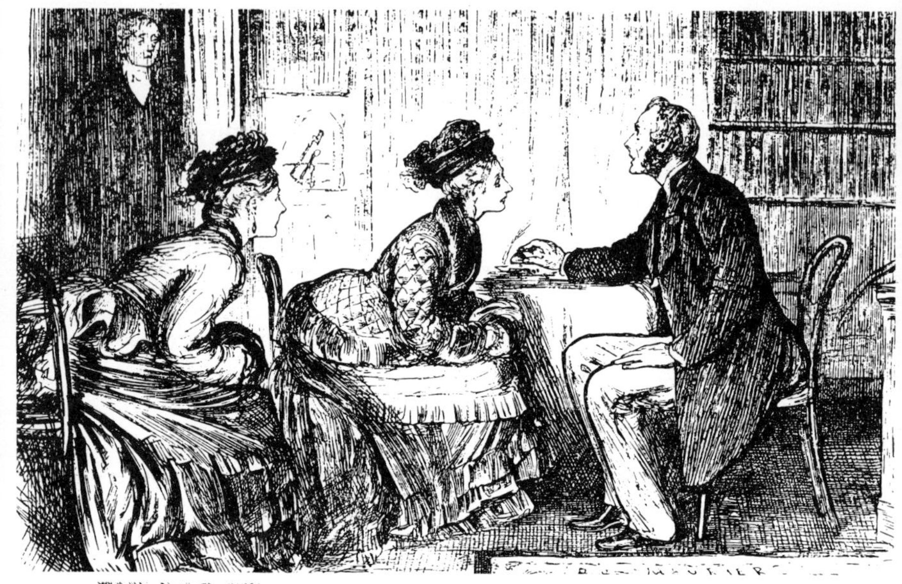

'THE EARLY BIRD CATCHES THE WORM' 1875

Struggling young Physician (who, after listening with rapt attention to the symptoms of his first patient, strikes a hand-bell and summons his faithful attendant) : 'OH, ER—ROBERTS!'
Roberts: 'YES, SIR.'
Physician : 'WHEN MR. GLADSTONE COMES, TAKE HIM INTO THE BREAKFAST-ROOM, AND ASK HIM TO BE SO KIND AS TO WAIT A LITTLE WHILE.'
(To Patient) : 'NOW, MADAM!'

The new doctor attends his first patient at his consulting rooms. In order to impress, he pretends he has another patient coming–Mr Gladstone, the Prime Minister!

pay him handsome fees. Such people expected attention from their doctor and he was at their beck and call. They did, after all, pay for each visit. If the doctor was good-looking and generally presentable he found himself attending patients–ladies mostly–who had little wrong with them but who thought it pleasant to have a handsome doctor sitting at their bedside–and well worth paying for. A doctor either had a good 'bedside manner' (in which case his practice increased), or a poor 'bedside manner' (when his patients left him). The doctor-patient relationship was very close. It was nice for a patient to be able to pour out her (or his) troubles to a sympathetic doctor who was expected to listen and make soothing sounds. Such confidences could not be told to friends or relations. One's secrets were safe with the doctor.

The expression 'family doctor' really meant what it said. He understood the difficulties of a family's life, each member of that family had probably confided in him at some time or another; he had possibly been present at the birth of all the children–and perhaps one of the parents.

The Victorian doctor had a double role: to attend families where there was specific illness, and to reassure in times of trouble and to give advice. As we know, some illness is due to a troubled mind, and today there are specialists to consult. A hundred years ago it was the family doctor who very often successfully treated such cases because he knew and understood his patient so well.

Although it must never be forgotten that doctors gave devoted service to rich and poor alike, the 'fashionable' doctor who was called in to give a 'second opinion' on a patient's illness, was sometimes a figure of fun. Charles Dickens, in 'Dombey and Son' gives a cruel little sketch of Dr Parker Peps who was anxious that everybody should know that he was consulted by the highest in the land. He had been called in by the Dombey's family doctor (or practitioner as Dickens calls him) who was greatly impressed by Dr Peps's fame and sucked up to him accordingly. The scene is Mr Dombey's house where his wife lies ill:

> ' "Well, Sir," said Doctor Parker Peps in a round, deep, *sonorous* voice, muffled for the occasion, like the knocker; "do you find that your dear lady is at all roused by your visit?" "Stimulated as it were?" said the family practitioner faintly: bowing at the same time to the Doctor, as much as to say, "Excuse my putting in a word, but this is a valuable connection." '

To Mr Dombey, Dr Parker Peps had this to say:

> ' "We must not disguise from you, Sir," said Dr Parker Peps, "that there is want of power in Her Grace the Duchess–I beg your pardon; I confound names; I should say, in your amiable lady. That there is a certain degree of *langour*, and a general absence of elasticity, which we would rather–not–"

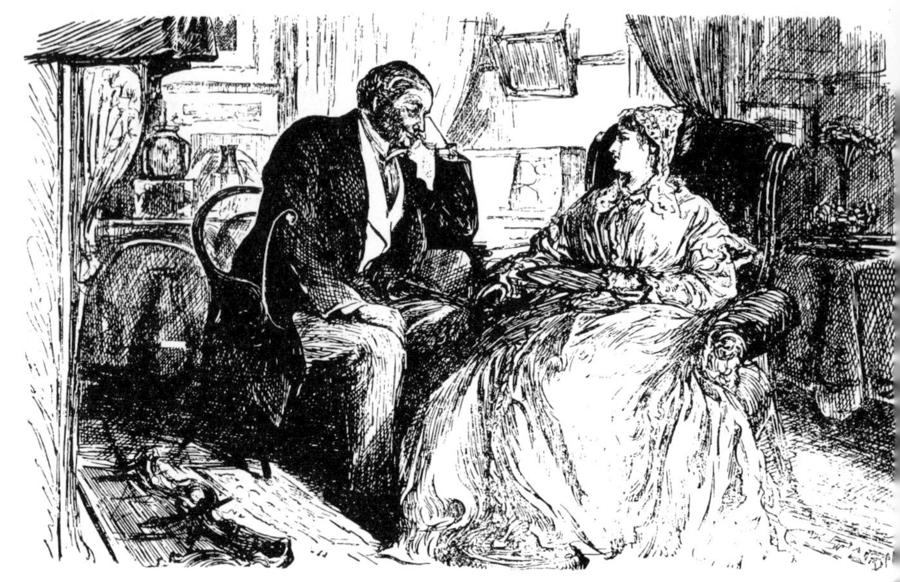

WISE IN HIS GENERATION

Fashionable Patient: 'COD-LIVER OIL!!! MY *DEAR* DOCTOR. I COULDN'T TAKE SUCH HORRIBLE STUFF AS THAT!'
Fashionable Doctor: 'WELL—WELL—WHAT DO YOU SAY TO—A—CREAM AND CURACAO?'

The doctor-patient relationship as seen by Punch. *A cosy chat. She doesn't seem very ill; he has all the time in the world. He suggests she takes cod-liver oil. When she throws up at the suggestion he substitutes cream and curaçao–a delicious liqueur! It really doesn't matter which she takes for her health! Notice his elegant clothes; he left his top hat in the entrance hall*

' "See," interposed the family practitioner with another inclination of the head.

' "Quite so," said Doctor Parker Peps, "which we would rather not see. It would appear that the system of Lady Cankaby–excuse me: I should say of Mrs Dombey: I confuse the names of cases–"

' "So very numerous," murmured the family practitioner–"can't be expected I'm sure–quite wonderful if otherwise–Doctor Parker Peps's West-end practice–"

' "Thank you," said the Doctor, "quite so . . ." '

'Keeping up appearances', 'wearing the correct clothes'–such things were important to the young doctor. A doctor who had achieved success was quite ready to give advice to younger members of the profession:

'Light-coloured clothing is dangerous for doctors because it will not stand soiling. . . . Nothing looks better on the head than a tall silk hat, anywhere. . . . Black boots should be worn on all occasions, never brown. . . . The London public demands a tall silk hat, as the doctor's head covering, and, make no mistake, this public will have it. . . . Light coloured vests or waistcoats may sometimes be worn to advantage.

'A walking doctor does not suggest the years of establishment that a driving one does; he may have just commenced, some people may think, and therefore he cannot be relied upon so instantly as the man who has rented stables and driven high steppers for years.

'One man I knew used to instruct his groom to drive up and down certain streets, so that people should think that he was attending somewhere near there.

'A certain doctor used to drive through his small town at break-neck pace once or twice a week so that people should think and remark, "Dr Enterprise must have several urgent cases: he seems to be sent for a great deal now." '

But in 1890 a book was published entitled 'The Young Practitioner, with Practical Hints and Instructive Suggestions as *Subsidiary* Aids for His Guidance on Entering Private Practice' by Jukes de Styrap, M.K.Q.C.P. (Member of the King and Queen's College of Physicians in Ireland) etc., Physician Extraordinary, Late Physician in Ordinary, to the Salop Infirmary (among other things). A glance through the index tells us a great deal:

'COMPANION, WHAT KIND TO SELECT: Let your *acquaintance* therefore be limited, as far as possible, to legitimate professional brethren and people of genuine worth. . . . At the same time, *eschew* the hotel bar, the smoking, the billiard, and the gambling room. . . .

'CREAKING BOOTS: The physician must tread softly. . . . I may note that for thirty years and more, it has been my rule to have a piece of sheet india rubber . . . inserted between the inner and outer soles . . . of my boots, with the signal advantage of not only thereby preventing them from creaking, but of keeping the feet dry in wet weather.

'FAMILIARITY, UNDUE: Frivolous conduct, vulgar jokes, great *levity* and *undue* familiarity are unprofessional. . . . Discourage all attempts to rudely address you with a "Hallo, Doc!"

'HABITS, DISGUSTING: You cannot be too careful in guarding against *repellent* habits, such as a breath reeking with the fumes of tobacco, spirits, beer, etc. . . . Moreover, to be seen carpentering, painting, or displaying other commonplace or out of place talents, will naturally lead people to *infer* that your mind is not so *engrossed* with your profession as it might and should be.

'SERVANTS, ATTENDING: Attendance on servants of the rich, however, especially if paid for by the latter, at the master's residence, will not *enhance* your reputation much. . . . People who, in their minds, associate you professionally with their servants, are apt to form a low opinion of your status, and the nature and class of your practice.

'TELEPHONE, THE: A telephone may . . . become a necessity, and even a luxury. Many practitioners, however, are *deterred* from having one by the fear that its convenience will lead to undesirable calls and messages at unreasonable hours.

'WHY CHARGE FOR EVERY VISIT: . . . let it be clearly understood that you charge for services not results, and must be paid for your attendance, even though the patient should die, and that all who seek your advice must accept the usual risks of cure or relief. Although, having accepted charge of the case you are morally bound, pay or no pay, to conscientiously fulfil your duty to the patient, you may, nevertheless, fairly intimate to those whose *pecuniary credit* you have reason to doubt that if they pay as they go on, it

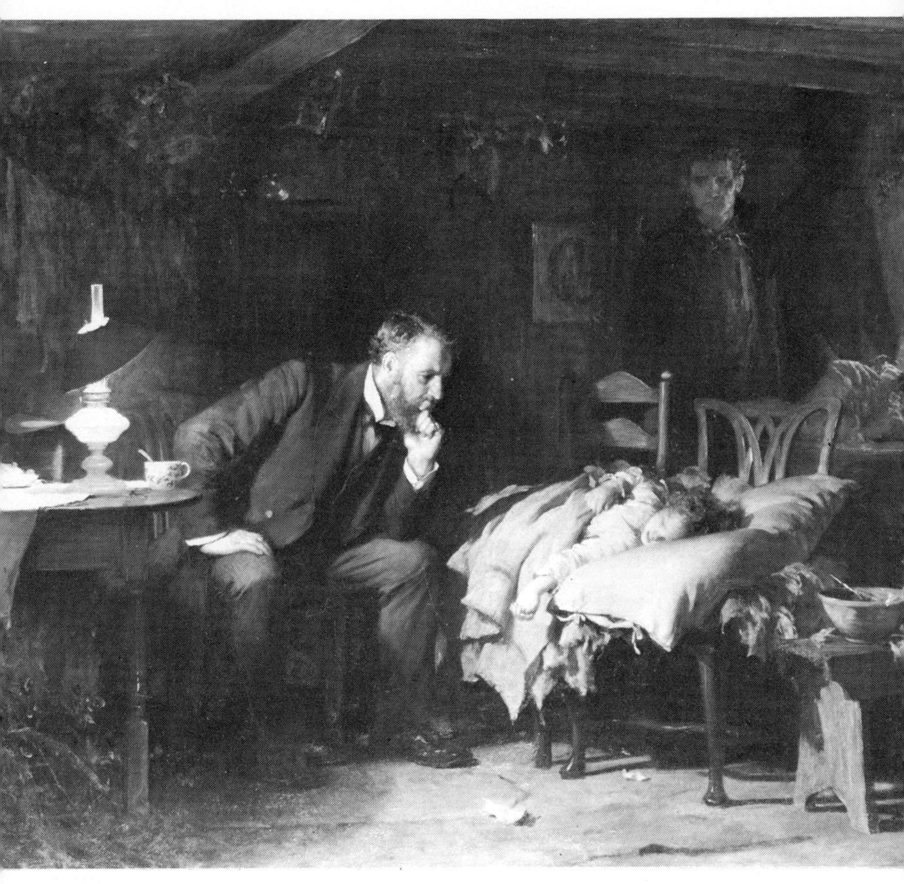

The Victorian doctor, far removed from the way Punch *saw him. He looks at the sick child not knowing what to do for her. In the background the mother buries her head in her arms; the father, grim faced, looks towards the doctor. This famous painting by Sir Luke Fildes, is in the Tate Gallery*

will tend to encourage and interest you more in the case, and naturally stimulate you to do your best.'

Much work done by the Victorian doctor he did for nothing or for little pay, but he had to live and his standard of living depended on the fees he received from his 'better-class' patients. You cannot blame him. This situation was typical of the age; it was the poor who got a rough deal.

7 *Medical Care for the Poor*

In 1598 Queen Elizabeth I passed a law compelling the people of each parish in England to provide for the poor and the sick. Before then the poor were nobody's responsibility unless a wealthy citizen tried to look after them. The Poor Law of Elizabeth's time protected the 'paupers' as they were called, from starvation, but they were looked upon by the more fortunate members of the community as an evil that had to be lived with. If paupers were to be cared for and restored to health, the food and shelter given them must be as little as possible and, when possible, the pauper who was fit to do so must earn his keep by working.

Elizabeth's Poor Law lasted over two centuries. In 1834 a new Poor Law came into force. Instead of paying money to paupers, they were made to seek help in a workhouse governed by a Board of Guardians. It was thought that if the workhouse could be made sufficiently unpleasant it would discourage people from applying for help. Only the destitute and sick entered the workhouse and as soon as they were well enough to be discharged, out they went. No parish wanted to keep paupers–they cost money and that led to an increase in the rates–so the unfortunate souls moved from parish to parish, or town to town, seeking help from any workhouse that would accommodate them.

Entry into a workhouse meant the end of family life. Husbands were separated from wives; children from mothers. The buildings were bare, gaunt, and crowded. Each workhouse had a master and a doctor, the doctor having less authority than the master. The master needed no qualifications for the job. He might have been ex-Army, or at one time have kept a cheap lodging house. The doctor – or medical officer as he was called – struggled on as best he could under very difficult conditions. He received little pay – possibly only £50 a year – out of which he generally had to supply all or some of the medicine needed.

In the Shoreditch Workhouse in London the Medical Officer had some 700 patients under his care of whom 220 were sick and 140 insane or subject to fits. He did not live in the building. He was 'wretchedly ill paid at the rate of £120 a year, is supposed to find an opportunity for performing adequately the medical service of this vast establishment in about two hours of morning visit, during which he has to perform the combined duties of medical officer, *dietist* and *dispenser*'.

Dr Joseph Rogers, in the latter part of 1854, was living in Soho in London. He had been in general practice for some ten years. An epidemic of cholera caused the death of so many of his patients that he hadn't got enough people to look after. He was offered the job of Medical Officer of the Strand Workhouse, Cleveland Street, Soho. 'Here I began,' he writes, 'my experiences of the sick poor, which lasted for thirty years. My first impressions were not very exhilarating, and could I have foreseen all that was in store for me, I question whether I should have applied for the appointment at all.'

He describes the workhouse: 'a square four-storeyed building fronting the street. Across the irregularly-paved yard in the rear was a two-storeyed lean-to building, with windows in the front only, used as a day and night ward for *infirm* women. There were sheds on each side for the reception of so-called male and female able-bodied people.'

He tells of an underground apartment lighted by a single window for the reception of paupers. 'The necessary laundry work of the establishment, which never in my time fell below five hundred inmates, was carried on in the cellar beneath the entrance hall and the general dining room . . . the said hall

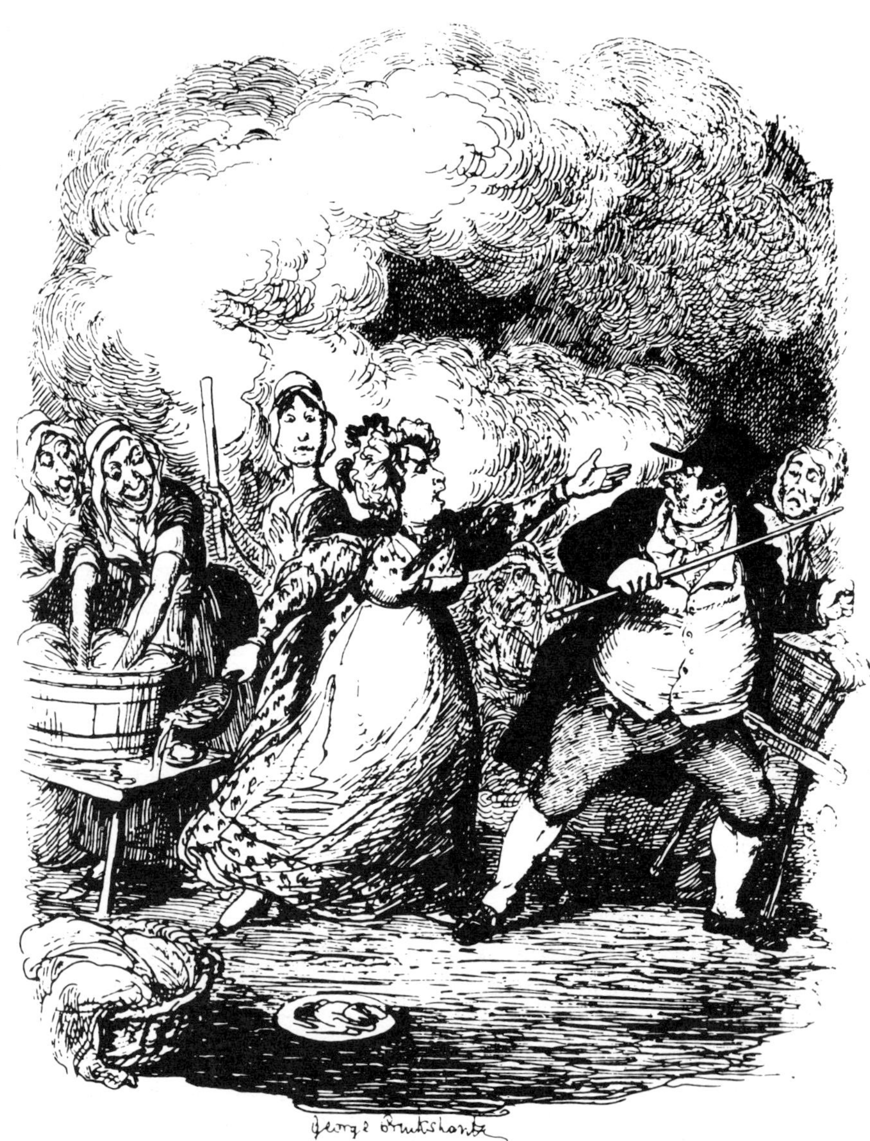

Mr Bumble in Oliver Twist, *master of the Workhouse (amongst other things) is seen here being told off by his wife in front of the delighted workhouse inmates. Drawing by George Cruickshank (1792–1878)*

etc. was for four days in each week filled with steam and the odours from washing the paupers' linen.'

Dr Rogers describes the carpet beating that used to take place just outside the male ward. 'The so-called able-bodied inmates' did the beating and the Board of Guardians was richer by some £400 a year. In spite of 'the continual noise and dust caused by this beating' it went on for ten of the twelve years he was there. 'The noise was so great that it effectually deprived the sick of all chance of sleep, whilst the dust was so thick that to open the windows was entirely out of the question until the day's work was done.'

The Chairman of the Board of Guardians was 'the proprietor of a beef-shop. This dignitary,' explains Dr Rogers, 'would often come to the [Work] House on Sunday morning dressed in the dirty, greasy jacket in which he had been serving the night before, and unshaven and unshorn, he would go into chapel with the pauper inmates, and afterwards go to the Board-room, and have breakfast with the master and the matron. Of course, between the three, there was an excellent understanding, and during this Chairman's reign all alterations for the better were resisted.'

Dr Rogers was sickened with the conditions. He describes the nursery ward which:

> 'was a wretchedly damp and miserable room, nearly always overcrowded with young mothers and their infant children. That death relieved these young women of their illegitimate offspring was only what was to be expected, and that frequently the mother followed in the same direction was only too true. I used to dread going into this ward, it was so depressing.'

The nurses were paupers. They received no pay; at times, perhaps, a glass of beer. 'Occasionally,' states Dr Rogers, 'for laying out the dead, and for other specially *repulsive* duties, they had a glass of gin.'

Dr Rogers tells of the time a Master left the Workhouse. 'So intensely tyrannical and cruel had been the rule of this man, that on the day he was leaving the whole establishment—at least all those who could leave their beds – rose in open rebellion, and with old kettles, shovels, penny trumpets, celebrated [his] departure from the premises.'

You can no doubt imagine these thin, pathetic, scraggy sick people, ill-clothed and dirty, with just enough strength to send the Master on his way, and it is not difficult to picture the expression on the Master's face as he strode down the wards on the way out.

Early in the twentieth century the workhouse was still a place to be avoided. There were improvements, but it was not until 1929 that the Board of Guardians was abolished and the duties handed over to the local authorities. The workhouse buildings were converted into hospitals, and the shame of being a workhouse inmate no longer applied.

Although the workhouse catered for the destitute who were ill, there was a large number of the population living in country districts who were miles away from any kind of hospital treatment. They were not necessarily destitute. A Dr Andrew Wynter, writing in 1866, summed up the situation:

> 'In large tracts of country there was no refuge to which poor creatures suffering from the terrible accidents on the introduction of steam machinery to agricultural pursuits and the railway, could be taken, but the Union Workhouse. Even in his own home imagine a poor wretch with a fractured leg, or some accident involving the nervous system, shut up in a single sleeping room of his cottage with noisy children to the *barbarous*, because *untutored*, nursing of his wife. If taken to the nearest Town hospital, perhaps twenty miles in a rough cart, the injury was necessarily aggravated, or a case requiring hourly attention, he could only get a visit once a day.'

In 1859 Mr Albert Napper organised the Cranleigh Village Hospital. It was the first of the 'Cottage' hospitals. By 1865 there were eighteen of them, and by 1880 there were 180. These hospitals served the country districts and some grew into big hospitals that exist today. They were run and financed by local people who were 'subscribers' meaning that they paid an annual subscription to keep the hospital going. Some of the Cottage hospitals were started with a legacy, or perhaps a wealthy man donated a large sum of money. The hospital itself was generally run by a small committee, which often included the parson. Doctors in the district could attend to their own patients in the hospital. But sick people could not get into these hospitals unless they had at least some money and a well-known person to recommend them.

The committees believed that the patient should have 'the privilege of being able to pay something, however small, according to his means, for the treatment he receives'. What patients pay, they said, 'is to be fixed by their employer, in conjunction with the manager of the hospital'. (It would seem that the patient himself had little, if any, say in the matter.) 'The sums paid are very varied, and range from 2*s* 6*d* to 21*s* per week for ordinary patients; domestic servants, when admitted on the recommendations of their masters, being charged a higher sum, varying from 5*s* upwards.'

As well as being able to pay something, a patient, before he was admitted, had to have a Letter of Recommendation signed by a responsible person or somebody connected with the hospital. Here, in part, are extracts from such a letter made out in favour of an imaginary person:

> 'LETTER OF RECOMMENDATION
> with which all Applicants must be provided, except in cases of severe accidents or sudden emergencies.
> I hereby recommend Jack Jones, aged 57, by occupation a labourer, as a proper person to be admitted into the hospital, and I consider him capable of contributing 2*s* 6*d* a week towards his maintenance. I further undertake to remove him when required to do so, and, in the event of death, to *defray* all funeral charges. Patients afflicted with *mania*, *epilepsy*, infections or incurable diseases, are *inadmissible*.'

Finally: 'It is requested that the persons sending the case will direct the patients to be sent as clean as possible, and with a sufficient change of linen.'

These Cottage hospitals were poorly but adequately furnished and from various sources we learn:

> 'Patent commodes which can be removed as required are preferable to a water closet, which in peasants' hands soon gets out of order.'
>
> 'Every properly administered hospital should provide these articles for the patient, and make him or his friends pay a certain deposit on them, to be returned when he leaves hospital.

	s	*d*
Small earthenware teapot		6
Cup and saucer		3
Two or three plates		4
Basin		2
Knife and fork	1	0
Tablespoon		3
Teaspoon		2
	2	8

> 'A cruet-stand and salt-cellar should be provided for the use of each ward. Very pretty cruet-stands can be made in fretwork. Should there be a lady or gentleman in the parish who does such work, two stands might be given to the hospital at almost nominal cost. They are easily fitted up with bottles at any glass shop.'

Not all Cottage hospitals survived. The one at East Grinstead closed in 1874 for the reasons given by the doctor in charge:

> 'In this district there are very many wealthy resident and land proprietors, but scarcely any volunteered to help me. I became weary of making these appeals to people who seemed to consider that, by contributing to the support of

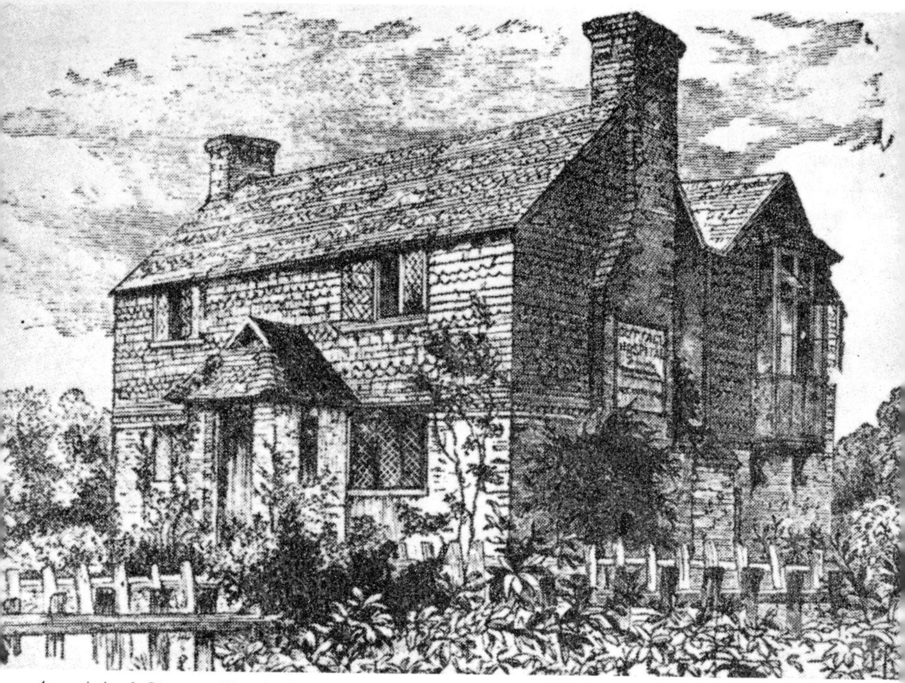

An original Cottage Hospital, Green Hedges, 1863, which grew into the Queen Victoria Hospital, East Grinstead, Sussex

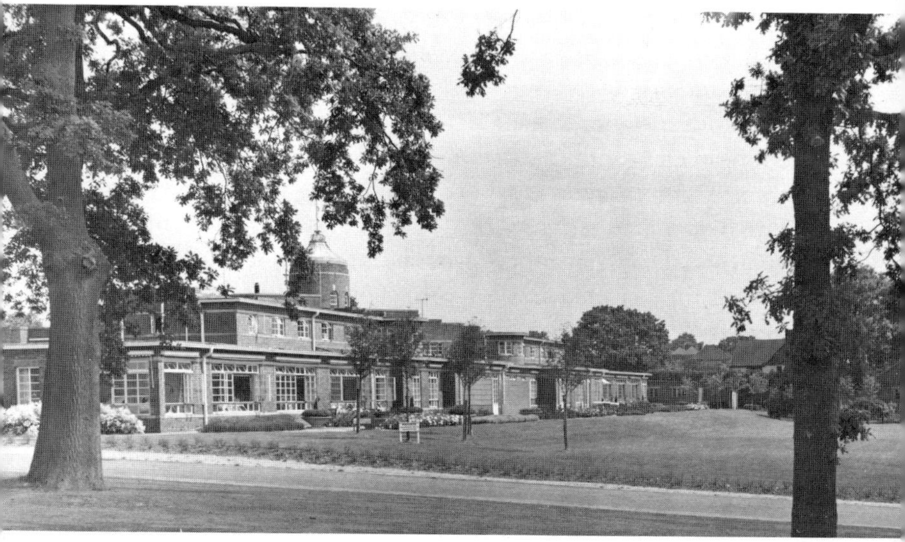

a hospital, they were conferring a favour upon me. In addition there were frequent attempts on the part of wealthy people to get their servants and dependants into the hospital so as to avoid paying towards their support. At length, after having experienced for some years the meanness of the wealthy, and too often the ingratitude of the poor, I closed the hospital.'

Despite this, a number of public-spirited wealthy people did contribute financially and gave their time to running these Cottage hospitals. The rules and regulations may seem harsh by today's standards, but many of them were necessary. The buildings were small and could not accommodate many. The patients were frequently dirty and dishonest. It was no fault of theirs. They had received little education and life was a struggle for them. Cottage hospitals–with all the restrictions–were better than no hospitals at all. The committees that ran them were anxious to do their best. The money came from people's pockets–not from the state. The committee members were, after all, Victorians–independent, God-fearing and stern. Those who received medical attention in their hospitals had to deserve it. We can see how they looked at the problem by two mottoes which a visitor saw as he entered the Boston Cottage Hospital. On one side of the entrance, the motto 'Rest and Be Thankful' was inserted in the brick wall, but on the opposite side were the words 'Work is Worship'.

Another source of help to the sick poor was the Medical Mission. The main work of the Medical Missions was in the then Empire overseas where the healing of the body was combined with preaching the Word of God. The missionaries visited tribes where there was sickness and no doctor to fight it except the Witchdoctor. A young physician fired with religious zeal thought he could do useful work among these peoples by restoring them to health and converting them to Christianity.

The missionaries thought that it was not only people abroad who needed the Word of God. In the poorer districts of Great Britain the 'ungodly' existed in vast numbers. There was work to be done close at home. A Medical Missionary

IF ANY MAN THIRST
LET THEM
COME UNTO ME AND DRINK
WHOSOEVER WI
LET HIM TAKE THE
WATER FREELY.
JESUS
ONLY
HALT
AVED
GOD
IS LOVE
IVE UNTO HIM
TERNAL LIFE
AND THEY SHAL
NEVER PERISH

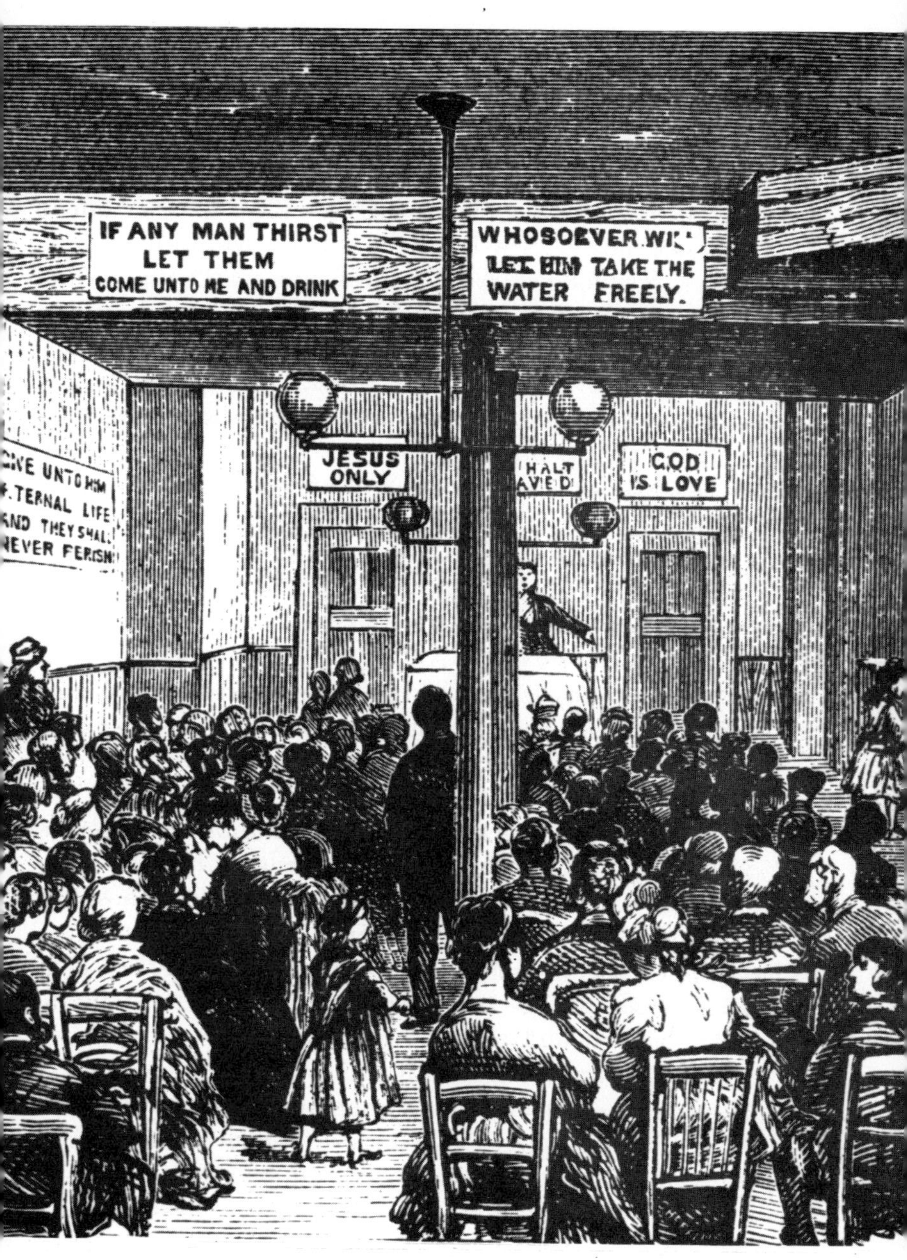

A Medical Mission. Prayers before the Pills

Dispensary was opened in Cowgate, Edinburgh at the end of the last century. An eye-witness describes the scene:

'It is the hour for the patients gathering. They come in dropping one by one. A pale, toiled-looking young mother, with a skinny, pining child. A heavy old woman in a faded shawl, with an expression of intense suffering in her brown wrinkled face . . . a lad with a hand wrapped up in a bloody *clout* follows. A tall, slim young man with the face of a consumptive, and dark eyes which almost glitter, coughs for some minutes, a cough hard and dry like the sound of an axe chopping wood. More mothers and children come in. What an effort these poor drudges have made to appear decently!

'Gradually the room fills with sufferers of every age and well-nigh every sort of ill. As the patients gather, a lady comes in, and sitting down among them, begins reading the Bible. To many of these poor patients, the word of God is absolutely a new sound.

'It is now two o'clock. A thin, work-worn man enters the room with an active, springy step, and his forefinger between the leaves of a Bible. It is Dr Burns Thomson, the Superintendent at the Institution. He looks round on his crowd of patients with a kindly smile and an eye which beams with benevolence. Opening the Bible he reads the words, "As Moses lifted up the serpent in the wilderness, even so must the Son of Man be lifted up, that whosoever believeth in Him might not perish, but have eternal life." He describes the camp of Israel–the working of the fearful serpent-poison, the convulsed shrieking wretches in the death agony, and all the horrors of the scene–and the picture he draws is so real it makes the flesh creep. . . . It was but a twenty minutes' sermon altogether, but so plain, so perfectly adapted to the class to whom it was spoken.

'A short prayer follows the sermon, and then the doctor retires to a separate room. The patients are shown in one by one.'

8 *Simpson and Lister*

Today, if we go to hospital for an operation, we are given an anaesthetic which puts us to sleep and we feel no pain. In the early part of the nineteenth century anaesthetics had not been discovered, and to have to undergo an operation was a terrifying ordeal. Here is a letter, written about one hundred years ago to a doctor, by an old patient:

> 'Before the days of anaesthetics, a patient preparing for an operation was like a condemned criminal preparing for an execution. He counted the days till the appointed day came. He counted the hours of that day till the appointed hour came. He listened for the echo in the street of the surgeon's carriage. He watched for his pull at the door bell; for his foot on the stair; for his step in the room; for the production of his dreaded instruments; for his few grave words, and his last preparations before beginning. And then he surrendered his liberty and, revolting at the necessity, submitted to be held and bound, and helplessly gave himself up to the cruel knife.'

The doctor who received this letter was James Young Simpson, a Scot born at Bathgate in Linlithgowshire in 1811. When, as a medical student, he attended an operation he was so appalled at what he saw that he seriously considered giving up medicine and studying law. The butchery in the operating theatre and the cries of the patients haunted him. How could this suffering be relieved?

In America, in 1844 and 1846, two dentists, Horace Wells and William Morton, had 'put patients to sleep' with ether and been able to extract teeth without the patients suffering

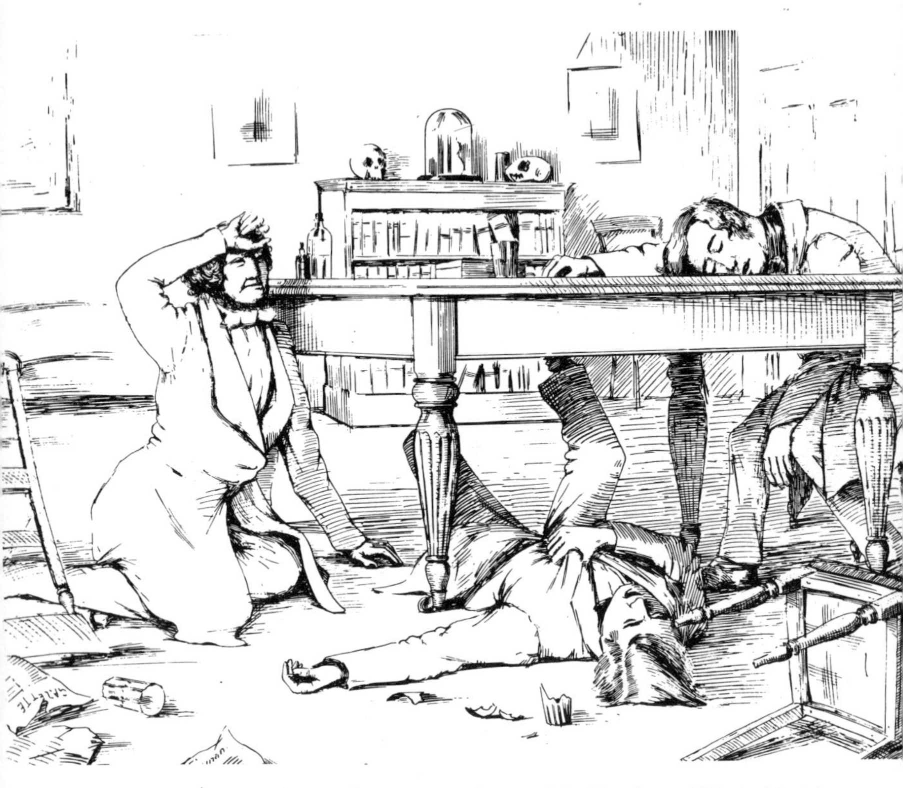

Simpson, left, and his colleagues, experiment with chloroform. This incident is described below

pain. This success prompted Simpson to carry out experiments. Ether had disadvantages and there is an account, by one of Simpson's neighbours and colleagues, of one night in November 1847 when Simpson returned home with his two friends and assistants, Drs Keith and Duncan. The three of them sat in the dining room and began inhaling various substances without much effect. 'It occurred to Dr Simpson to try a small bottle of chloroform.' The three men inhaled it and fell asleep. Dr Simpson was the first to wake.

' "This is far stronger and better than ether," said he to himself.' His friends were still asleep, 'Dr Duncan beneath a chair–his jaw dropped, his eyes staring, his head bent half under him; quite unconscious, and snoring in a most deter-

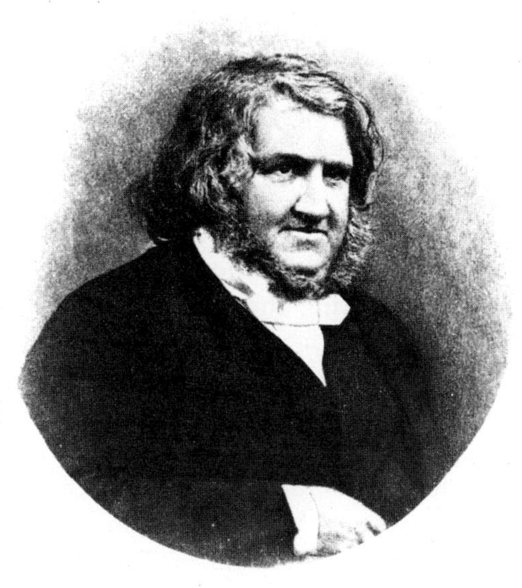

James Young Simpson who relieved suffering by the use of chloroform. As a medical student in the operating theatre, he was so horrified at what he saw that he nearly gave up medicine

mined manner.' Dr Keith was also asleep although his feet and legs were very active 'making . . . attempts to overturn the supper table'. On waking, each expressed himself delighted with chloroform and it was used in operating theatres thereafter.

Surgery ceased to be so horrific. Surgeons could work at a slower pace and with more care knowing that the patient was not suffering. The frightful butchery disappeared. Even so, there were those who opposed the use of chloroform for medical and religious reasons. Since Simpson's day other doctors doing research on this problem have found other substances which are used in appropriate cases. The giving of anaesthetics in an operation is a skilled job and some doctors specialise in this branch of medicine. The first doctor to do so was John Snow who administered chloroform to Queen Victoria during the births of Prince Leopold and Princess Beatrice. It was not until 1853 that Queen Victoria's Physician wrote to Simpson:

> 'That the Queen had chloroform exhibited to her during her late confinement [the birth of Prince Leopold]. It acted admirably. It was not at any time given so strongly as to render the Queen insensible, and an ounce of chloroform was scarcely consumed during the whole time. Her Majesty was greatly pleased with the effect, and she certainly has had a better recovery. I know this information will please you, and I have little doubt it will lead to a more general use of chloroform in Midwifery practice . . .'

This was a great triumph, for if the Queen approved, everyone else was sure to do so. Sir James Young Simpson as he became, was acclaimed throughout the world, and after his death in 1870, a marble statue was erected in St Andrew Chapel, Westminster Abbey in his honour:

'To whose genius and benevolence
The world owes the blessing derived
From the use of chloroform for the
relief of suffering.
Laus Deo'

Another hazard in the first half of the nineteenth century was dirt. Nobody recognised its danger. There is the story of a famous surgeon, Sir Astley Cooper, who was called to his patient, King George IV (reigned 1820–30). On arrival Sir Astley's hands and shirt were stained with blood from an earlier operation he had conducted. His Majesty viewed his doctor's appearance with a certain amount of distaste and when the stains were pointed out, Sir Astley remarked, 'God bless my soul! I was not aware of it; and the King is very particular.'

In the hospital wards and operating theatres the opportunities for washing were limited. Jugs of water, basins and towels were there for washing hands and instruments, but the

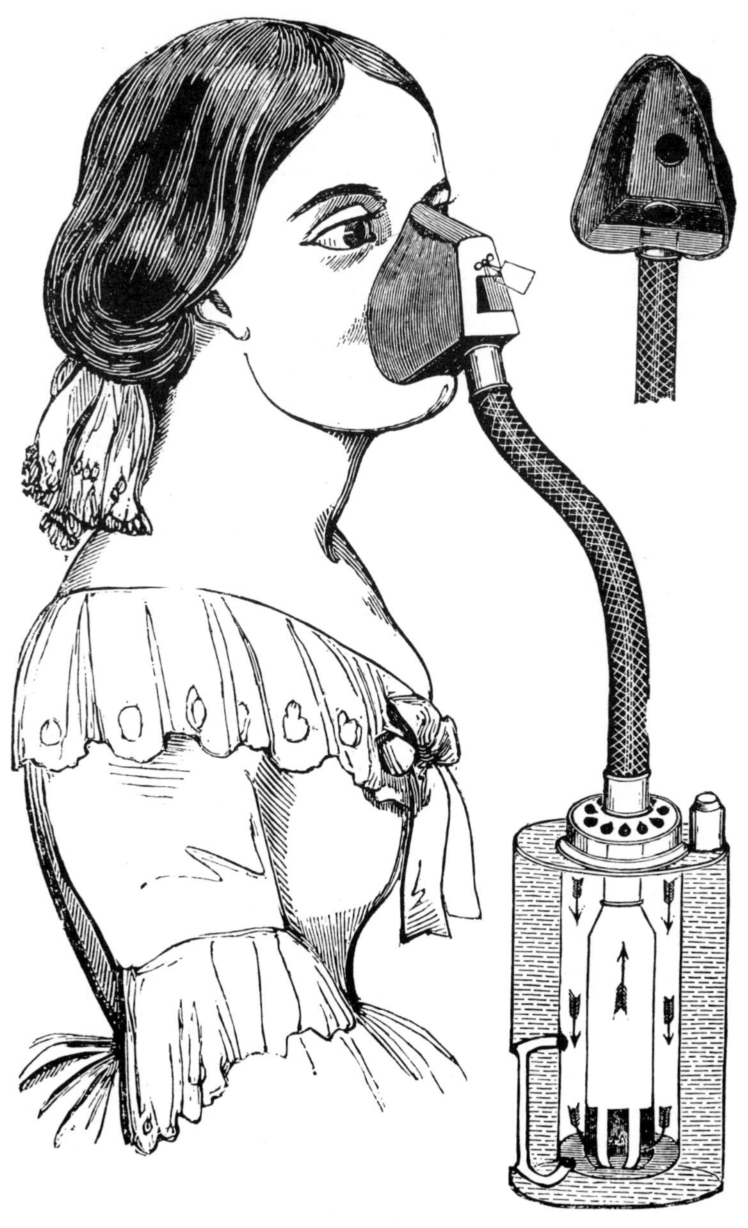

How chloroform was given in the 1850s. The lady looks wide awake!

former were generally washed after the operation rather than before, and the latter received a mere rinsing before being used again.

Surgeons, doctors, dressers, wore their ordinary clothes. In fact the old coat, stained and filthy, was often kept in the operating theatre, just as a city clerk keeps a patched jacket for work at his desk. Doctors, surgeons and nurses passed freely from the dead to the living, carrying infection with them. The results were disastrous. The chances of survival in a surgical ward were slim; one out of every three patients died. In military hospitals the percentage of deaths was even higher–75 to 90 per cent.

On a spring morning in 1865 a doctor by the name of Joseph Lister stepped from his carriage which had drawn up outside the gates of the Glasgow Royal Infirmary. Into the building he carried a sample of carbolic acid and it was this disinfectant he used to kill germs. He had experimented over a period of time, working far into the night, as to how carbolic acid could best be applied. It was Lister's belief that germs entered wounds from the hands of a doctor or surgeon, the instruments and dressings, and from the air in the operating theatre.

The famous French scientist Louis Pasteur (1822–95) had done brilliant research on germs and their effect, and Lister was the first to acknowledge his debt to the Frenchman. 'We find', wrote Lister, 'that a flood of light has been thrown upon this important subject by the writings of Louis Pasteur.'

Now, when he operated, Lister removed his coat, rolled up his sleeves and, to protect his clothes, pinned a large towel over his trousers and waistcoat. He washed his hands and dipped them into a strong solution of carbolic acid. His instruments lay in the same disinfectant. Then he set to work.

Lister also invented a device which sprayed carbolic acid into the air thereby destroying germs. At first the spray was worked by hand and if the operation took a long time relays of assistants were needed to keep it going. Later a spray was developed that worked by steam.

Joseph Lister was born in 1827 at Upton (then an isolated village) in Essex. His father was a Quaker from Yorkshire. He had a happy childhood with brothers and sisters, and his choice of career was entirely his own. There had been no doctors in his family before. As his fame increased, so did his popularity. He was worshipped by his students, and to have been associated with Lister even in a humble capacity was a great honour. Lister did not write about himself; only his work. It was left to his friends and associates to proclaim what a great man he was.

Joseph Lister's carbolic spray in use during an operation. Notice that the surgeons wear their everyday clothes

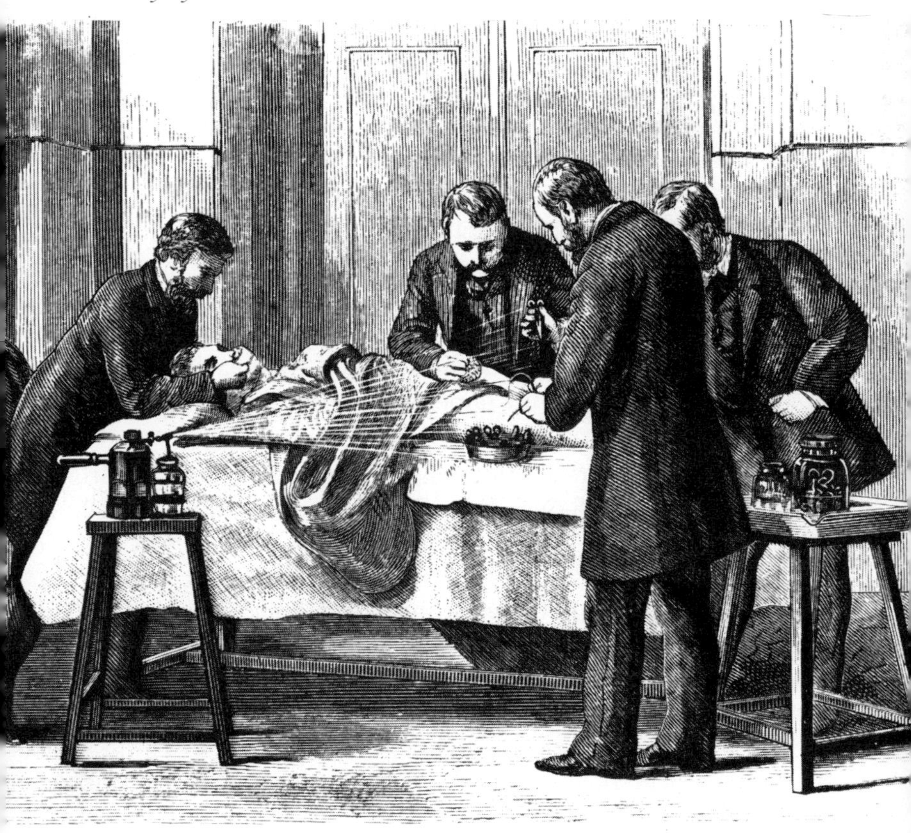

A Canadian associate of Lister gives this picture of Lister visiting an Edinburgh hospital:

> 'It is the old reserve ward for men and about two o'clock on a summer afternoon. Clerks and dressers and some students from other clinics are standing about chatting together or talking to the patients. The instrument clerk in charge of the famous spray is seated on the broad window sill at one end of the ward for the spray must be kept ready for instant use. Then someone suddenly says, "Here comes the Chief" and we see our hero come through the little side gate down the slope with his easy, rapid stride. . . .
>
> 'I wonder if there were anywhere else in the world a surgeon whose pupils held him in more reverent admiration or whose patients trusted him so. It was his wish on Sunday to see every patient in his wards. He goes from bed to bed, occasionally conversing with a patient or discussing a case with the House Surgeon but never using a word to alarm or distress a patient.
>
> 'And so through all the men's wards, then downstairs to the women and children. How their eyes follow him! And perhaps the visit ended in the famous little ward at the back, in which were two big beds. In one, three small boys, Tommy Miller, Roden Shields and Willie Shotts, all "chronic" spinal and joints, doomed to early death or at least deformity and lameness but for him–all happy and recovering.'

The use of antiseptics–since developed from the original carbolic acid–originated by Lister was a startling success. An operation was no longer a likely death sentence. On the continent, especially in Germany, Lister's discovery was enthusiastically adopted. Only Britain held back. Those who had taken the trouble to study what Lister was doing, became converted to his ways. Lister's work had been done in Glasgow and Edinburgh, but it was only when he came to London and worked there that people realised the importance of antiseptics.

Lister was the first medical man to be created a peer. He died in 1912 just before his eighty-fifth birthday. There is a

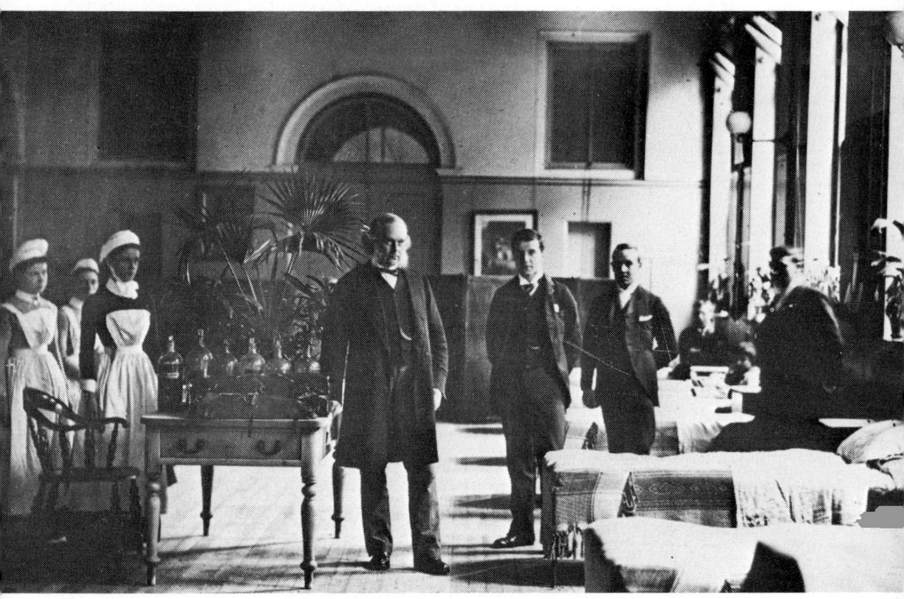

Joseph Lister, the central dominating figure in the photograph. It was taken in 1890 in a ward of King's College Hospital, London

medallion of him in Westminster Abbey and he is buried with his wife in the West Hampstead Cemetery, London.

There have, of course, been other great medical discoveries in the last hundred years or so. Almroth Wright (1861–1947) introduced anti-typhoid inoculation and did research on vaccine. Alexander Fleming (1881–1955) with Howard Florey and E. B. Chain discovered penicillin, but Joseph Lister must surely be regarded as one of the leading benefactors of humanity. The number of lives saved through the use of antiseptics cannot be counted. In fact the entire history of surgery falls into two parts–before Lister and after Lister–and the contrasts have been explained in this chapter.

Coupled with Lister's name must be Simpson's, whose use of anaesthetics relieved suffering that before his time was sometimes more than the human body could bear.

9 The State Takes Over

'Take the utmost care to get well born and well brought up. This means that your mother must have a good doctor. Be careful to go to school where there is what they call a school clinic, where your *nutrition* and teeth and eyesight and other matters of importance to you will have been attended to. Be particularly careful to have all this done at the expense of the nation, as otherwise it will not be done at all, the chances being about forty to one against your being able to pay for it directly yourself, even if you know how to set about it. Otherwise you will be what most people are at present: an unsound citizen of an unsound nation, without sense enough to be ashamed or unhappy about it.'

GEORGE BERNARD SHAW, writing in 1911.

You have read how the poor received a raw deal when it came to medical attention. Some people contributed a few pennies each week to a Friendly Society, and when they were ill the Society met the doctors' fees. But it was a haphazard arrangement. When things were bad the weekly payments stopped. Consequently much of the population could not afford to be ill. A doctor was often called when it was too late.

Towards the end of the nineteenth century many influential people were thinking along the lines of National Insurance. This meant that the state should be responsible for the welfare of the sick and that medical attention should be made available to those who could not afford it. In 1880 an association was formed for the purpose of educating and informing public opinion on the subject of National Insurance. People who were keen on this idea wrote about it in important magazines.

In the early years of this century statesmen in the Government began to think about it and Lloyd George, a fiery Welshman who at that time was Chancellor of the Exchequer in the Liberal Government under the Prime Minister Herbert Asquith, took a keen interest.

'Never was legislation more needed,' said Lloyd George and 'never was it less wanted.' The plan was that the worker, his (or her) employer and the Government should contribute a sum of money each week, and the worker would be placed on a doctor's list or 'panel' as it was called then. The worker became a 'panel' patient and was entitled to medical treatment without payment. This is the basis of the National Health Service as we know it today, but sixty or so years ago it did not do nearly as much as it does now.

All sorts of people opposed Lloyd George. The doctors were suspicious because it meant that the state controlled them to some extent; the Friendly Societies were suspicious because their usefulness was threatened; and those not in need of free medical treatment objected because the scheme was too kind to the poor. It was a form of socialism and not to be tolerated.

There were months of arguments, meetings, protests, but the National Insurance Act took shape. 'I never said this Bill was a final solution,' said Lloyd George at Birmingham in the summer of 1911. 'I am not putting it forward as a complete remedy. It is one of a series.' He likened himself to the driver of an 'Ambulance Wagon'.

> 'I am engaged,' he continued, 'to drive a wagon through the twistings and turnings and ruts of the Parliamentary road. There are men who tell me I have overloaded the wagon. I cannot spare a single parcel, for the suffering is very great. There are those who say my wagon is half empty. I say it is as much as I can carry. Now there are some who say I am in a great hurry. I AM rather in a hurry, for I can hear the moanings of the wounded and I want to carry relief to them in the alleys, the homes where they lie

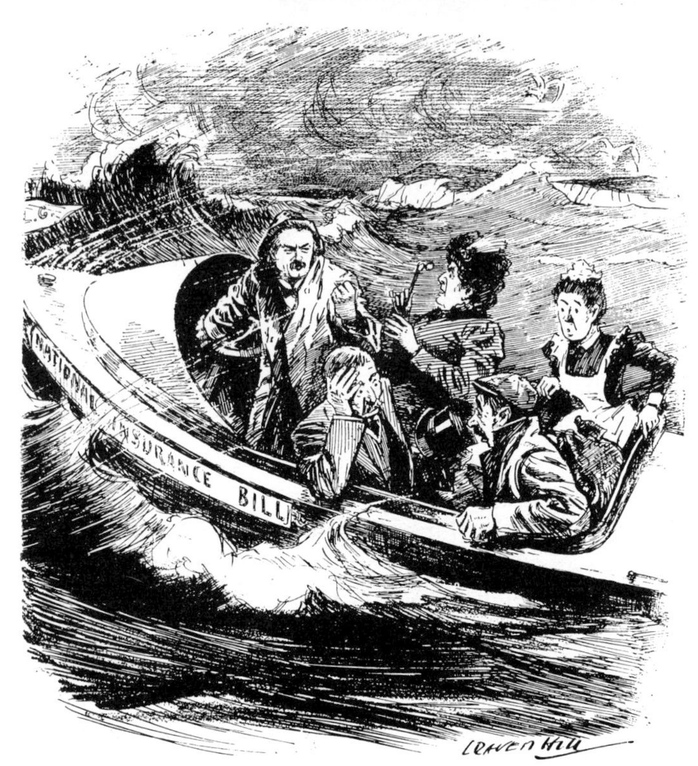

THE PITILESS PHILANTHROPIST.

MR. LLOYD GEORGE. "NOW UNDERSTAND, I'VE BROUGHT YOU OUT TO DO YOU GOOD, AND *GOOD I WILL DO YOU*, WHETHER YOU LIKE IT OR NOT."

The National Insurance Bill, 1911. Lloyd George (in sou'wester) takes an unwilling cross-section of the public for a rough ride

> stricken, and I ask you, and through you I ask millions of good-hearted men and women – the majority of people in this land – to help me set aside hindrances, to overcome obstacles, to avoid the pitfalls that beset my path.'

Mr Bonar Law of the Conservative opposition thought that the Ambulance Wagon was 'more like a motor car careering downhill with broken brakes'. Eventually Lloyd George came to terms with the doctors. In some respects the doctors in poorer districts did well. Their patients were often bad payers and now the doctors were assured of an income of 9*s* per person on the 'panel'. The Friendly Societies had not been left out of the scheme and public opinion was also in favour.

The Insurance Act became law in December 1911. King George V had just been crowned.

The Act was in two parts – one part relating to health and the other to unemployment benefits. Part 1 – the health part – laid down that all workers in regular employment between the ages of sixteen and seventy, not earning more than £160 a year had to contribute 4*d* a week; his (or her) employer 3*d* a week and the state 2*d* a week.

In return the worker was entitled to enrol on the 'panel' of any doctor who agreed to take him into the scheme, and he received free medical attention. The worker would also receive sickness benefit varying from 5*s* to 10*s* for men, and from 3*s* to 7*s* 6*d* for women for a period of twenty-six weeks, but this would be followed if necessary, by a disablement benefit which normally amounted to 5*s* a week. A maternity benefit of 30*s* was available. All these benefits, however, were only granted to the insured worker and not to his or her family. Hospital services were free only in cases of real poverty and it was necessary to show the authorities that you were in need.

What use, you may think, could these very small benefits be to anybody? In 1912–13 in four medium-sized industrial towns, a third to a quarter of the adult workers were earning less than 24*s* a week. In 1913–14 the average adult earned 30*s* for a working week of fifty-four hours. So you will realise that a benefit of even 3*s* was worth having, while 10*s* must have seemed a princely sum.

Cards were issued to all employers and stamps had to be stuck on to them. Aristocratic ladies very much objected to having to lick the stamps for their servants. Spurred on by the 'Daily Mail' of that day, the Servants Tax Resisters Defence League was formed and some 20,000 women inside and outside a meeting at the Albert Hall cried: 'We won't pay. Taffy was a Welshman, Taffy was a thief.' (Taffy meant Lloyd George who was Welsh.) Of course, said certain sections of the public, the money paid in benefits to the deserving poor would be wasted. Those of you who know 'The Charge of the Light Brigade' will appreciate this rhyme:

'THE CHARGE OF THE SICK HUNDRED

With the money to pay the rent
Which Lloyd George had kindly lent,
Happy sick hundred!
And though they are badly crushed,
Into the pub they rushed,
Later with faces flushed,
Homeward they went.'

But in spite of the 'Daily Mail' and the objections of the few, everybody paid up, and employers have been sticking stamps on cards ever since. Aristocratic ladies, in times of illness, had two doctors to their house. Their own private doctor whom they paid, and the 'panel' doctor for the servants, paid by the state. He was taken to the servants' quarters at the top of the house by the housekeeper.

After the 1914–18 war against Germany, the National Insurance Act was improved, but it still did not do nearly enough. It was during the 1939–45 war that the National Health Service, as we know it today took shape.

In 1941 Mr Ernest Brown, Minister of Health in Winston Churchill's Coalition Government, announced the decision to create a national hospital service after the war. In 1942 Sir William Beveridge (as he then was), a brilliant administrator who had worked out rationing systems at the outset of the war, produced what came to be known as the Beveridge Report in which he recommended a comprehensive health service.

The Report was issued at a time when Great Britain's fortunes were at a low ebb. We were engaged in a desperate war against Hitler's Germany and nobody knew how long it would last, and it was difficult to be sure of the outcome.

The Beveridge Report, therefore, was an act of faith for the future. It was, said Beveridge, 'a completion of what was begun a little more than thirty years ago when Mr Lloyd George introduced National Health Insurance'. The Report was widely cheered. It sold 635,000 copies–unheard of for a

KINGSLEY WOOD & Co
COATS TURNED
SUITS THAT FIT (US)
NO TURN-UPS—POCKETS UNNECESSARY
BESPOKE TAILORING
(NOT FOR THE TROOPS)
BRITISH PEOPLE

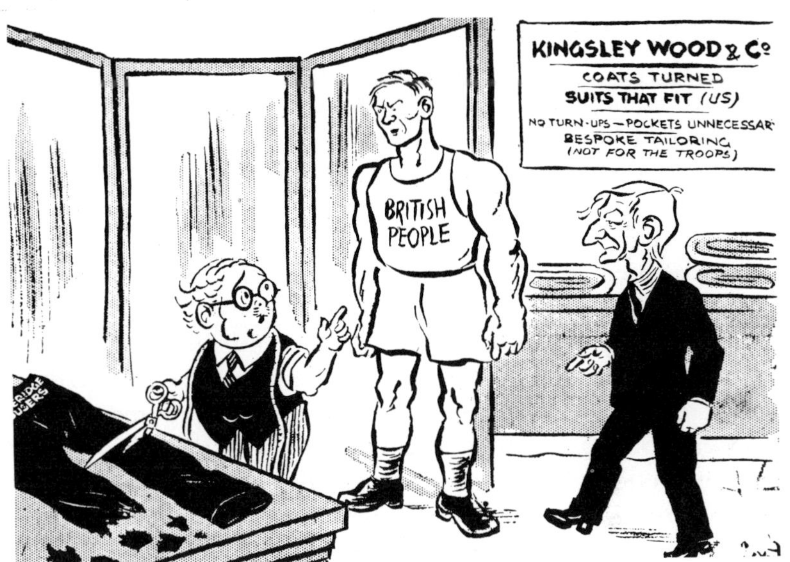

The Beveridge Report. Beveridge (right) watches his social service plan (shown in the cartoon as 'Beveridge trousers') being cut down by Kingsley Wood who was Conservative Chancellor of the Exchequer in the National Government. The man, representing the 'British People' looks on anxiously because by the time the scissors have been at work the 'trousers' aren't going to fit him. The Conservatives were unhappy about the cost of Beveridge's social service plan and were anxious to cut it. This cartoon, by the late 'Vicky' appeared in the News Chronicle *(now part of the* Daily Mail*) on 5th March 1943*

Government publication. Its content was discussed by those at home and those fighting overseas.

Sir William had this to say about it. It set out to make sure first:

> 'That no one in Britain willing to work while he can, suffers from want while for any reason–of unemployment or sickness or accident or old age–he cannot work or earn . . . that no man leaves his wife and children in want after his death. . . . My Report proposes . . . a unified social insurance system under which by paying a single weekly contribution through one insurance stamp everyone will be able to get all the benefits that he or his family [the 1911 Act only benefitted the insured worker] need so long as they need them.'

Second:

'A scheme of Children's Allowances so that all parents have enough to keep their children strong and healthy, and can have more children, if they want them without *stinting* the children they have already.'

Third:

'The plan proposes a comprehensive health service, securing medical treatment of all kinds for all citizens in return for the insurance contribution.'

In February 1943 the Coalition Government accepted the Report and set about planning the Health Service. At that period of the war Britain's fortunes were improving, but a Report so *controversial* was bound to meet with opposition. The main objection was the cost. Could we ever afford it after the war had ruined us financially? The Labour Party realised that it was a plan for social justice and they feared the Conservatives in the Coalition Government might want to water it down.

Another fiery Welshman, Aneurin Bevan, who was to become Minister of Health in the first Labour Government after the war said: 'The Beveridge Report, which was the one egg laid for post-war planning, the Tories are now doing their best to addle.' In July 1945 there was a General Election and Labour swept into power. On the crest of the wave was the National Health Service Bill, based on the Beveridge Report, which became an Act in November 1946. It was Aneurin Bevan who piloted it through. Like Lloyd George he met with objections from the various medical bodies. Reasonably enough, they had views as to how the service should be run and the content of the Act is the result of give and take on both sides.

How does the National Health Service work? The central administration is in the hands of the Secretary of State for Social Services. (There is no longer the title Minister of Health). He is advised by a Central Services Council of some forty members consisting of doctors, people with hospital management experience and others with experience of local government. Dentists, Mental Health experts, nurses, chemists, midwives are also represented.

The doctors get paid a sum of money for each person they attend (as they did for those on the 'panel' in the 1911 Act). The dentist, chemist, optician receives a fee for each service he performs, the patient making some contribution to the cost.

For hospital and specialist services there are Regional Hospital Boards which, with the Secretary of State's approval, offer guidance and are responsible for planning and control.

In each district there is a Local Executive Council, some of the members being appointed by the Department of Health and Social Security. This Council assists doctors and dentists and other medical men in the area to make the Health Service function. It publishes lists of medical men willing to take patients and it pays the doctors who are in the scheme. It also deals with complaints.

Lastly the local authorities are responsible for maternity and child welfare services, district nurses, home helps, ambulances, after-care.

A doctor may have Health Service patients and also attend patients privately who pay him, but whether or not a patient makes use of the Health Service, he has to contribute to its cost.

Lloyd George did not live to see the 'final solution' to his National Insurance Act of 1911. He died in March 1945. It was left to his compatriot, Aneurin Bevan (who died in 1960) to bring about the final solution in the form of the Health Service as we know it today. 'The essence of a satisfactory Health Service,' said Bevan, 'is that the rich and the poor are treated alike, that poverty is not a disability, and wealth is not advantaged.' Lord Beveridge (as he became) on whose Report the Health Service as we know it today is based, died in 1963 at the age of eighty-four.

A far cry, indeed, from the dark years of the nineteenth and early twentieth centuries.

10 *The Health Service: Performance and Problems*

Have another look at the cartoon on page 77 which shows Beveridge's social service plan being 'cut'. There have been more 'cuts' over the years and we have not been able to do all that Aneurin Bevan hoped for the Health Service when he wrote the words at the foot of page 79.

The cost of running the Health Service, the provision of medicines and drugs, pay for doctors, surgeons, consultants, nurses, hospital staff became so high that the insurance payments were not providing enough money and the Government needed to cut down expense.

The medicines the doctor says a patient should take have (with exceptions) to be paid for partly by the patient although it does not cost him or her anything to consult the doctor. People under sixteen years of age, however, and old age pensioners do not have to pay for medicines prescribed by a doctor. Beveridge had hoped that our insurance contribution and general income tax would pay for all medical care, including medicine.

Some people argue that charging for medicine is wrong. They say that because people know they will have to pay for the medicine the doctor prescribes they do not go to the doctor. This might mean that their illness might become worse.

Other people say that when all medical care was free people went to the doctor much too often for pills and medicine. Now that pills and medicine have to be paid for people do not go so often, and that is all to the good!

In the cities and big towns doctors are often overworked. Their surgeries are sometimes in old buildings, the rooms small and cramped. The building of health centres has made things easier for doctors. The health centre was first mentioned in an official report in 1920, but it was not until the National Health Service Act of 1946 that local authorities were called upon to build health centres, and it was not until the 1970s that a great many health centres were built.

A health centre is exactly what the name suggests. Doctors get into a group to run a health centre. There they can see their patients in pleasant surroundings. Patients are shown into nicely-furnished waiting rooms. Health care can be given, for example, to children, expectant mothers, old age pensioners. Patients, who before this had to go to hospitals for treatment, can now be treated at the health centre. The doctors share the services of receptionists who make appointments and look after medical records. Nurses working at a health centre can give treatment under the doctor's orders. Specially-trained health visitors run baby clinics where mothers bring their babies to be weighed and to get advice.

So throughout Britain health centres make better working places and pleasant places for patients to come to, while all the things doctors need are under one roof. But not all doctors are convinced that health centres are a good thing. Some feel, rightly or wrongly, that a health centre is less 'personal' (and some patients feel that way too) because it is run by a local health authority and doctors are not so free to do what they think best.

Some people do not make use of the Health Service. They prefer to see a doctor privately and pay him a fee. If they need an operation they prefer to go to a nursing home where they can have a bed in a private room. They do this because they believe they are receiving more personal attention. An operation performed by a surgeon of their choice can be done at a convenient time; they may not have to wait.

Some doctors, surgeons and consultants work within the Health Service and also see 'private' patients who are prepared to pay them. Nurses and other staff trained in Health Service hospitals then get jobs in private nursing homes. This, some

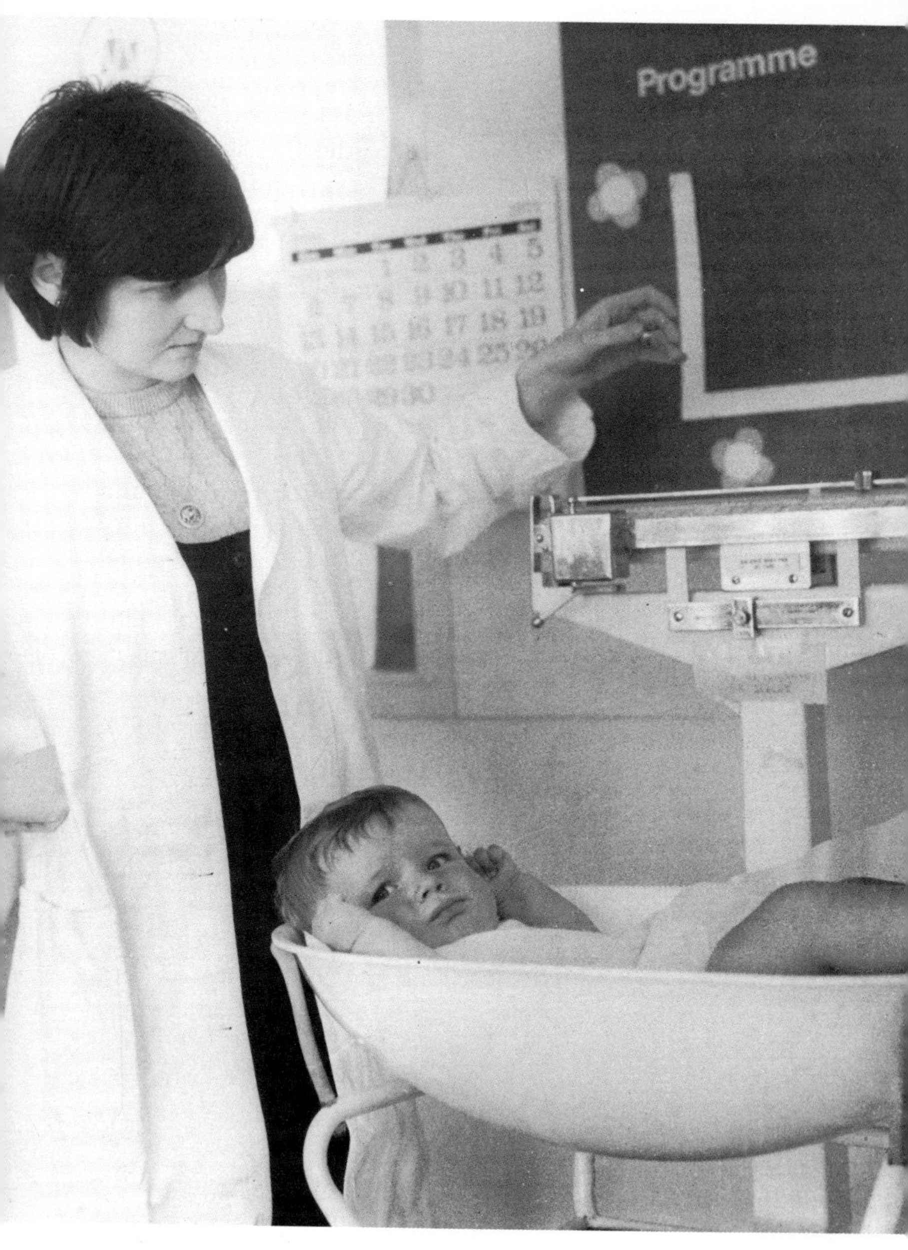

 Child care at a Health Centre

people say, should not be allowed to happen.

Some big hospitals where Health Service patients go have a wing where 'private' patients are catered for. These 'pay beds', as they are called, can cost the patient over £100 a day plus what has to be paid to the doctor, the surgeon and for medicines.

Despite the protests about pay beds there is a growing demand for them, not only from the wealthy but from those with modest incomes. How can such money be afforded?

There are organisations which will contribute to your medical expenses if you pay them a certain sum of money each year. It is a form of insurance; the more you pay, the greater the contribution towards your medical expenses. Many industrial companies 'insure' their employees in this way. When employees need hospital treatment they can go 'privately' and their medical care is paid for. Although many want private medicine, some people think it is unfair to those who cannot afford it, and that it takes away good staff from the Health Service.

George Bernard Shaw wrote: 'Do not try to live forever. You will not succeed.' True enough, but people today do often live longer. This is due to medical research, 'preventive' medicine (see below) and because we live healthier lives.

In 1851 the population of the United Kingdom was about 22 million. In the 1980s it is well over 50 million–more than double. The United Kingdom has not got any bigger and yet room has been found for all those extra people! Why, then, are there no cholera epidemics which were caused by crowded housing in the nineteenth century? The answer is because everything is cleaner. Our food comes packaged and clean although it has lost much of its flavour in the process. Food manufacturers and food shops have to obey strict rules in the preparation and the selling of food products. We drink pure water. Milk is 'pasteurised' (the treatment of milk is based on Louis Pasteur's discoveries). The air we breathe may be free from smoke although we do inhale petrol fumes. Refuse is collected and the drains are flushed. So despite the fact that there are many more of us than there were a hundred years ago everything is done to make sure that we are kept in good health.

'Preventive' medicine means preventing people from having illnesses and diseases, or treating them at an early stage so that the trouble does not get bad. At one time tuberculosis (known as 'TB' or 'consumption') affected the lungs and could be passed from one person to another. Now it is no longer a danger due to our better living, to the pasteurisation of cow's milk and the regular examination of people by X-ray which reveals the disease at an early stage. Children are *inoculated* against whooping cough, measles, *diphtheria*, polio and TB. Babies are tested for their hearing, and examined to see if there is anything wrong with them. If there is, this can often be put right if discovered early enough.

This 'preventive' medicine can be done at the health centres. The discovery by Sir Alexander Fleming and others of *penicillin* and *antibiotics* have made it possible to cure illnesses which used to kill people.

In Victorian days the noise in factories was terrible and the unguarded machinery was often very dangerous. People worked from dawn to dusk six days a week and they were paid a tiny wage at the end of it. People lived packed together in cities. Sanitation was hardly known. There was no preventive medicine. You only entered hospital when you were very ill. The wards were crowded, the beds perhaps made of wood and bug-infested. Can you imagine how people got ill in their minds because of all the strains and stresses of life a hundred or more years ago? They were so poor and life was so hard. Remember Florence Nightingale's pitiful cry: '... but if something is the matter with the MIND it is neither believed nor understood.'

If you were a woman a hundred years ago you were often stopped from having a busy and interesting life. You might not be allowed to go to college and rich girls had too little to do. Elizabeth Garrett reminds us that she was 'living at home with nothing to do. I was full of energy and vigour and of the discontent which goes with unemployed activities . . .' For the sick mind a chat with the family doctor might help a little, but for poor people little was done. They would be dumped in *asylums* and forgotten.

The wealthy, up to the 1914 War, ate immense meals and could be said to have dug their graves with their teeth. The poor were underfed and they–as well as the rich–drank too much beer and spirits.

Today we work reasonable hours and have the good holidays denied to the workers in Victorian times. *Mental illness* is recognised, treated and often cured. People get sick in their minds for different reasons, not because life is poor and hard but because it goes too fast and people compete so much against each other. Noise is not only in factories. Cars, lorries, aircraft are all noisy. Frightening accidents on the roads cause injury and death. The Victorians at least did not have these troubles.

We eat well but not so much as the Victorians did. We do not always eat sensibly although we should know what is good for us. We are lazy. We watch sports on television rather than take part in them. We are always munching something and in some respects we are as bad as the Victorians. Consequently we become too fat and what is known as *obesity* is a health problem.

There is too much drinking today. In Victorian times people drank to forget their troubles. Now people drink because it is the 'smart' thing to do, and intoxicating liquids can easily be bought by the young who, by law, should not be able to get them. Too much drink makes for bad health in later life. Those who take to drugs are also damaging their well-being.

As far back as 1858 Florence Nightingale said that hospitals should not be in towns. Town air was not pure enough, she wrote, and existing town hospitals ought to be removed to the country. All that was needed in town and city centres were a few casualty wards and after examination the patients should be transferred 'in suitable vehicles' to hospitals in the country. How prophetic! She saw what we are doing now.

Hospitals are being moved into less crowded areas. More and more people are moving out of the cities and towns–they like to live outside them–so hospitals can be built in pleasant places where there is space to expand. Industry is also moving out of the cities into places where it is cheaper to rent offices and factories can be healthier for employees.

Although new hospitals have been and are being built, there are too many still in old buildings where wings have been added and corridors wind like snakes from one wing to the next. 'Temporary' outside buildings have been put up which become 'permanent', and covered passageways, cold and draughty, lead to them. It is surprising that such good medical care can go on in such old buildings.

New hospitals being built have special parts planned to take the *chronically ill*, the mentally ill and those suffering from special diseases. The hospital becomes a 'community' consisting of a number of buildings different in size and shape, each planned, equipped and staffed according to the medical needs of the patient. 'Preventive' medicine, as we have seen, is of growing importance. The object is to keep people out of hospital, but it must be possible to perform difficult surgical operations if required.

Everything is being done to keep us fit and happy. Take a look once more at the William Hogarth picture on page 27. We have come a long way since then, and we should remember Florence Nightingale, James Simpson, Joseph Lister, Alexander Fleming and many others with gratitude.

Things to Do

1. Write an imaginary conversation about plans for the future between Florence Nightingale at the age of seventeen and a girl of the same age today.
2. Find out as much as you can about the Crimean War: why it was fought and where and what the results were.
3. Write a letter home from a wounded soldier describing Florence Nightingale and her nurses at work in the hospital at Scutari.
4. Write a letter to the *Times* arguing the case for having a State Register of Nurses. Then write a reply by Florence Nightingale (p. 23).
5. Discuss in class whether Florence Nightingale or Elizabeth Garrett had the harder struggle to fulfill her ambition.
6. Write down all the ways in which you think the life of a modern doctor differs from that of a Victorian doctor.
7. Discuss in class why people allowed the workhouses described in chapter 7 to go on for so long.
8. Find out if there is (or has been) a Cottage Hospital in your district, and, if so, who started it and how it was paid for.
9. Write and act a scene in which Drs. Simpson, Keith and Duncan try out the effects of chloroform on themselves (see p. 64).
10. Find out more about the lives of Louis Pasteur and Joseph Lister. You could use an encyclopedia for this.
11. What have been the greatest medical discoveries in the twentieth century? Make a list of these.
12. Write an imaginary speech by Lloyd George in support of the first National Insurance Act in 1911.
13. Hold a class debate on the good and bad points of the National Health Service today.
14. Visit the Wellcome Museum of the History of Medicine at The Science Museum, South Kensington, London SW7, where medical history is fascinatingly displayed.

Glossary

abbreviation, shortening
accomplice, workmate in crime
acquaintance, person(s) one knows slightly
alacrity, cheerful readiness
alpaca, woollen cloth made from llama's hair
anaesthetics, drugs to make people unconscious during operations
anatomy, structure of the body
antibiotics, substances capable of injuring or destroying living organisms, especially useful in medicine for destroying bacteria which cause disease
antiseptic precautions, care to prevent germs entering wounds (antiseptis — against poison)
apothecary, skilled medical chemist (word no longer used)
arrowroot, West Indian plant from which flour is ground to make a nourishing drink for invalids
asylum, a home or hospital providing care and safety for the mentally sick
audacity, boldness
avarice, love of money
barbarous, rough, unskilled
besets, surrounds
chaperones, older women who used to accompany girls not allowed out alone
chronically ill, people who suffer constantly from some kind of serious disease which cannot be cured
clout, cloth
compact, close together
comport, behave
confinement, birth of a baby (the mother being 'confined', i.e. kept in bed)
controversial, giving rise to argument
cordial, friendly
courier, travelling attendant able to speak foreign language(s)
cul-de-sac, road closed at one end
defray, pay for
delirium, a disturbed mind

deterred, held back
dietist, one who advises on suitable food
diphtheria, a very infectious disease, chiefly of children. The symptoms are a severely inflamed throat, heart and nervous system
dispenser, one who makes up and gives out medicines
dissipation, frivolous entertainment
dresser, (dressings) person to attend to wounded and apply bandages
egg-flip, drink made of egg beaten in milk with spirits (e.g. rum, whisky) or wine added
engrossed, fully occupied
enhance, improve
entertain, here means 'consider'
epidemic, a disease spreading to many people at one time and place
epilepsy, a nervous disease causing fits
eschew, avoid
faculties, abilities
fomentation, bathing with warm water
forenoon, morning, before noon
genial, kindly, sociable
gruel, nourishing drink made from oatmeal
gruesome spectacle, horrible sight
inadmissible, not allowed in
infer, come to the conclusion
infirm, sickly, unwell
ingenious, skilful
ingrained, thoroughly known, given importance
inoculate, to bring about a mild form of a particular disease, by injecting someone with the micro-organisms which cause it, as a safeguard against future infection
keep, here means board and lodging
languor, lack of energy
Laus Deo, praise God (Latin)
leech, bloodsucking worm that used to be much used in medicine
levity, lightheartedness
mania, madness
mantle, cloak
medallion, here means an inscribed stone fixed to the wall
mental illness, a sickness or disorder of the mind
nutrition, food to keep the body healthy
obesity, unhealthy fatness
pallet, straw mattress
pecuniary credit, money in hand, ability to pay

penicillin, a mixture of substances produced by certain types of mould which is able to prevent the growth of some kinds of disease-carrying bacteria
post-mortem, medical examination after death
poultice, soft wet pad, usually hot, applied to a wound
probationer, nurse under training
repellent, unpleasant, putting off
repulsive, disgusting
sanitation, services to protect health, especially drainage
sonorous, loud-sounding
squat, low
stinting, depriving
subsidiary, additional
superfluous, more than enough
swabbing, washing
tedious, boring
thoroughfare, through road
Tsar, emperor, head of Russian state before the Soviet revolution
undue, excessive
untutored, untaught
veneering, a thin layer of good material laid over less good (often used in carpentry)
ventilation, circulation of fresh air